What People Are Saying about *The Diarrhea Dietitian*

"I thought I knew everything after seeing multiple dietitians and dealing with both ulcerative colitis and Crohn's disease over the last 9 years, but this book proved me wrong. Whether you have Crohn's, ulcerative colitis or IBS this easy-to-read book will help make life more livable. It is full of methods to ease diarrhea not only from evidence-based research, but also from wisdom that only comes with years of working as a GI dietitian."

~S.R., BSN

"Whilst overwhelmed with the task ahead– working out how to reduce the diarrhea nightmare–this book will give readers likely understandable causes to this problem. It will also give them the motivation to start tackling it in a more informed, logical way rather than just hoping one day it will all go away. I recommend partners, family members, and friends of the sufferer also read the book to develop a greater understanding of the complexity of this condition, and to be able to offer more empathy and support to the person to begin and travel on this journey."

~J.R. (Sydney, Australia)

"Niki Strealy, The Diarrhea Dietitian, is acutely aware of the problems clients face living with complicated bowel issues. In her book, you can feel her personally guiding you through the topics with a level of understanding that is easy to relate to. She gives the reader the tools they need to adapt their lifestyle and ease complications. This is a usable and very 'real' resource for clients' personal use as well as dietitians, nurses and doctors working with individuals that struggle with diarrhea."

~S. Wood, MS, RD

The Diarrhea Dietitian

Expert Advice, Practical Solutions, and Strategic Nutrition

Niki Strealy, RD, LD

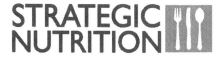

x

Lake Oswego, Oregon

The Diarrhea Dietitian: Expert Advice, Practical Solutions, and Strategic Nutrition

http://www.DiarrheaDietitian.com/
niki@DiarrheaDietitian.com

Strategic Nutrition, LLC
P.O. Box 2013
Lake Oswego, OR 97035

ISBN: 978-0-9889793-4-5

Printed in the United States of America

This book is dedicated to all of you who belong to the

Secret Diarrhea Club.

May this book get you out of the bathroom, and back into life.

Table of Contents

Acknowledgments

Thank you to my patients, for reminding me how many people out there are limiting their lives because of diarrhea. This book is for you!

Thank you to my parents, family, friends, and co-workers, for letting me talk about diarrhea again and again...even in the lunchroom or at the dinner table.

Thank you to my awesome sister Angie, whose graphic design talents never cease to amaze me. You put aside your projects to help me finish mine; I am both grateful and humbled.

Thank you to my pharmacist team, for using your clinical skills to help me. Uncle John, you rock at chemical equations! Dan, I miss working with you on the metabolic support team. Thank you both for reviewing the medications chapter.

To my awesome team of reviewers: Sydney, Susan, and Jenny, I appreciate your comments, suggestions, and honesty in helping me to make this book truly relatable for everyone. To Patsy Catsos, thank you reading through my manuscript and expanding my knowledge of FODMAPs. You have been so kind to share your knowledge on self-publishing. I am very grateful.

Lastly, thank you to my husband Alden and three favorite kids, Aidan, Ethan, and Audra for sacrificing time with me so I could finish this manuscript. I absolutely could not have completed this task without your support...and many trips to the library so I could work alone. Thank you for believing in me.

Introduction

Good News

Is diarrhea affecting your quality of life? Your job? Your relationships? Are you afraid to leave the house? Is it preventing you from going on vacation? Exercising? Taking a class? Attending an outdoor sporting event where there aren't bathrooms nearby? In short, is diarrhea preventing you from really living your life?

Regardless of whether or not you have been given a specific diagnosis, this book can help you gain control of your diarrhea and get back to doing what YOU want to do.

Diarrhea is a Dirty Word

When you're sliding into first and your pants are going to burst, diarrhea cha-cha-cha, diarrhea cha-cha-cha. When you're sliding into home and your pants are full of foam, diarrhea cha-cha-cha, diarrhea cha-cha-cha.

You may have heard children chant this silly song before. The truth is, if you are one of the millions of people affected by chronic diarrhea, this is no laughing matter. No one wants to hear, much less talk about, diarrhea. That's why we use slang words like the trots, the runs, green apple quickstep, Hershey squirts, and Montezuma's revenge. Can you think of others?

When I first told my friends and family I was writing this book, it was amazing to hear the different comments. Some were too embarrassed to talk about it at all. Others wondered, "Who would want to read a book like that?" My favorite response is, "Well, if YOU had diarrhea and couldn't talk about it, wouldn't you be glad to find a book you could read instead?"

Even the medical community has found it hard to assess how many people actually have chronic diarrhea in the United States. Studies have indicated that it may be as many as five percent of the population— upwards of 15 million Americans! Chronic diarrhea can be debilitating and isolating; many people are afraid to leave the house for fear they won't make it to the bathroom in time. Others are unable to maintain employment because of the need for frequent trips to the toilet.

As a registered dietitian, I have observed similar behaviors in those with chronic diarrhea. I call this group "the secret diarrhea club." There are millions of fellow sufferers, yet no one knows each other. They know the location of every bathroom in town and often carry an "emergency diarrhea kit."

Are you in this club? Here are some clues:

- You know every bathroom location in town (this is called bathroom mapping)
- When you go in a bathroom, you always check the toilet paper supply and maybe even carry your own

- You have your own emergency kit in the car or at work, containing toilet paper, unscented baby wipes, extra clothes and 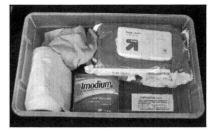 underwear, anti-diarrheal medication, and barrier cream

A Little Bit about Me

I started experiencing diarrhea in my early teens. Due to a family history of ulcerative colitis, I underwent my first barium enema at age 13, followed by a small bowel follow-through and sigmoidoscopy by age 17. Since they never found anything clinically wrong with me, my doctor shrugged his shoulders and labeled me with irritable bowel syndrome or IBS.

My friends and family have always known about my ongoing diarrhea episodes. I decided long ago not to keep it a secret. I nicknamed it "Mr. D" so could tell a story without embarrassing people who were unable to hear the word without cringing.

Like many of you, I have experienced diarrhea at the most inconvenient and embarrassing times and places: during church, at restaurants and school, during sporting events, concerts, while exercising, on dates, airplanes, and road trips. Sometimes my body gives me plenty of time to find a bathroom, other times not nearly enough.

On one occasion, when I was a sophomore in high school, I had a soccer game about an hour's bus ride from my home town. After the game, the bus was just beginning the drive home when the first diarrhea cramp hit. I soon realized that I wasn't going to be able to wait an hour before needing a bathroom. I made my way to the front of the bus to explain to my coach why we needed to stop. I must have looked desperate, because she made the driver pull the school bus (filled with 35 girls) into the nearest gas station. After spending 45 minutes in the restroom, I finally got back on the bus and was greeted by a standing ovation!

Later in high school, I went to the county fair with a group of friends. Once again, the diarrhea urge was coming. By the time I got to the restroom on the other side of the fairgrounds, there were at least 10 people in line ahead of me. Just when I didn't think I was going to be able to wait any longer, a stall opened up and I started to walk inside. At the same moment, a woman with a little girl burst into the restroom and pushed her way into my stall, breathlessly telling me I needed to wait because her little girl was going to have an accident. Little did she know I was about to have one too! To this day, I don't know how I managed to wait until another stall opened up a few minutes later.

Due to my early experiences, I became fascinated by the anatomy and physiology of the human body, especially the gastrointestinal (GI) tract. I remember coloring my digestive diagrams in high school elective anatomy class. I began college as a pre-med student, but was drawn to nutrition science. More specifically, I was interested in how food is processed and absorbed through the intestines into the body. After graduating with a degree in Nutrition and Food Management, I completed the required one-year internship.

The dietetic internship trained me to teach patients to follow diabetic, renal, weight loss, weight gain, surgical, and other diets, with little emphasis on gastrointestinal diets. But as I began my career as a registered dietitian (RD), it became my passion to educate patients on how and what to eat for their digestive problems.

For several years I worked in hospital critical care and surgical units, seeing a lot of people with Crohn's disease, ulcerative colitis, gastric bypass, and cancer surgeries. Since 2002, however, I have focused on outpatient nutrition counseling, specializing in GI diseases and disorders. My professional training and personal experiences with chronic diarrhea have given me a unique understanding of and empathy for what my clients are going through.

Before We Begin

My first recommendation is to visit your primary care provider and describe your symptoms. You may want to read ahead to Chapter 19: Discussing Diarrhea with Your Doctor. Be assertive—do not be afraid to give details about your bowel movements. You may be referred to a **gastroenterologist**, a physician who specializes in the identification and treatment of digestive diseases and disorders. Your doctors may put you through a series of tests. You may be given a diagnosis, or you may be told, "We can't find anything wrong with you."

The Plan of Attack

This book covers the anatomy and physiology of the GI tract, food digestion, and how the foods you eat impact the frequency of your bowel movements. We will cover many other topics, including the effect of stress on the gut, probiotics, medications, specific conditions, diseases, disorders, and food allergies and intolerances. I will also give you suggestions on what you CAN eat!

Unfamiliar medical terms, in **bold**, are defined at the end of the book in the **Glossary of Terms**.

While you can read the book straight through, word-for-word, *feel free to skip sections and chapters that do not apply to you!* The more you read, the more you will realize how complex a simple word like "diarrhea" can be. Each person is unique. You may find certain foods that you tolerate, while others do not. That is perfectly fine.

What Is Your goal?

For over 16 years, I have successfully helped my patients decrease their diarrhea, as well as reducing my own episodes, primarily through diet and lifestyle modifications. This has both given me freedom and improved my overall quality of life. This is my goal for you too! Let's begin this journey together.

Niki Strealy, RD, LD
The Diarrhea Dietitian

Chapter 1

Let's Get Started!

I know you are anxious to get rid of your diarrhea! In the medical field, all potential treatments are ideally subjected to a **randomized controlled trial (RCT)**. Unfortunately for those of us with diarrhea, there aren't enough of those studies available. It is both challenging and expensive to conduct studies on people with intestinal problems because there is so much variability. In addition, many studies are funded by drug companies. No one wants to pay for studies based on diet alone.

The table on the next page is a summary of my recommendations to stop, reduce, or alleviate chronic diarrhea. We will be covering these concepts in greater detail in subsequent chapters. These recommendations are derived from medical studies, professional observations, individual patients' case histories (called anecdotal evidence) or from my own personal experiences.

Not every point will apply to you, but I suggest moving through the list while trying only one suggestion at a time. Think of yourself as both the study participant and the control subject. If you change too many things at once, you won't know what worked. It may be helpful to record food intake and bowel movements in a journal for a week prior to trying any of these suggestions (see Appendices A and B). After making changes, refer back to your journals to see how your symptoms have changed.

Niki's Top Strategies to Stop Typical Chronic Diarrhea

Strategy	Read More in Chapter
1. Determine if you have lactose intolerance. Try a lactose challenge.	**4, 10**
2. Determine if you have fructose intolerance. Fructose is a type of sugar. Cut back on very sweet or rich foods and desserts.	**4, 10**
3. Minimize insoluble fiber intake. Try the Easy-to-Digest Diet in Appendix C. Soluble fiber is allowed.	**4**
4. Avoid sugar-free gum, candy, and medications that contain the sugar alcohols sorbitol, mannitol, or xylitol.	**4, 10**
5. Cut back or eliminate anything that contains caffeine, including coffee, tea, soda, chocolate, energy drinks, or diet pills. Caffeine makes everything in the intestine move through faster.	**4**
6. Limit intake of acidic, spicy, or high-fat foods, which can aggravate diarrhea.	**4**
7. Limit intake of alcohol-containing beverages. Alcohol stimulates the bowel and causes gas.	**4**
8. Manage your stress through exercise, prayer, yoga, meditation, massage, acupuncture, biofeedback, or hypnotherapy.	**7**
9. Take a probiotic as directed on the bottle for at least three to six months.	**8**
10. Discuss your medications with your physician or pharmacist to determine if any are aggravating diarrhea.	**9**
11. Try taking loperamide (Imodium®) as directed on the box.	**9**
12. Avoid bulk-forming fiber supplements such as Metamucil® or Citrucel®, which often exacerbate diarrhea.	**9**
13. If you have irritable bowel syndrome or inflammatory bowel disease (IBD), you may benefit from a low-FODMAP diet.	**10**
14. Get tested for celiac disease (CD), a digestive disorder that damages the small intestine and interferes with absorption of nutrients from food. Treatment for CD requires a lifelong gluten-free diet. Gluten is found in wheat, rye, and barley.	**12**
15. Consider medical evaluation for food allergies, bile-acid diarrhea, or small intestinal bacterial overgrowth (SIBO).	**13, 14, 16**
16. Take calcium supplements. Most people do not consume enough calcium, and it's constipating.	**17**
17. If you have been told you are anemic or need more iron, take iron supplements. They are constipating too.	**17**

Chapter 2

Basic Nutrition, Normal Anatomy and Physiology of the GI Tract: What Goes in Must Come Out

Before we discuss digestive anatomy, it is important to understand the main components in our food. Then we can review how the body mechanically breaks down and absorbs these important nutrients.

Food Composition Basics—Macronutrients

Your food is comprised of three important **macronutrients**:

- Carbohydrates
- Proteins
- Fats

Not all foods contain all three macronutrients. For example, some are a combination of protein and fat (meats such as beef) or contain only simple carbohydrates (such as fruits).

Carbohydrates

Carbohydrates are your body's most important energy source; they can be either simple sugars or complex carbohydrates. Simple sugars are found naturally in foods such as fruits, vegetables, milk, and milk products. Complex carbohydrates include whole-grain breads and cereals, starchy vegetables, and legumes.

The body breaks down carbohydrates from long chains into their simplest form called glucose, which the body uses for energy. The glucose is absorbed into the bloodstream, and is either used quickly or stored in the liver and muscles for later use.

Proteins

Proteins are important for the growth and maintenance of bones, organs, hair, skin, and especially muscle. They are also an important component of enzymes, hormones, and blood cells. The

> Including protein foods at meals and snacks provides *satiety*, or the feeling of fullness, after you eat. This explains why snacking on empty carbohydrates such as chips and crackers just make you feel hungry only a few minutes later!

body breaks down proteins into simpler building blocks the body can use, called amino acids and peptides (several amino acids linked together in chains).

In the diet, proteins come from plant-based foods (nuts and legumes, which are also complex carbohydrates) or animal products (beef, poultry, seafood, eggs, and dairy products).

Fats

Fats, also known as lipids, have the following functions:

- Provide energy
- Aid in absorption of fat-soluble vitamins A, D, E, and K
- Cushion and protect your inner organs

Fats also make your food taste better and improve texture. Not all fats are alike, however. **Trans fats** and **saturated fats** increase the risk of cardiovascular disease. In contrast, unsaturated and polyunsaturated fats may improve blood cholesterol, decrease risk of type 2 diabetes and cardiovascular disease, and lower blood sugar and blood pressure.

What percentage of my calories should come from carbohydrates, fats, and proteins?

Calories are the sum total of food energy provided by carbohydrates, fats, and proteins. Scientists and experts in the field of nutrition recommend a balanced distribution of calories in the diet to promote good health, about 55 to 60 percent carbohydrates, 15 to 20 percent protein, and 25 to 30 percent fat. The following chart shows the optimum calorie distribution for each of the macronutrients.

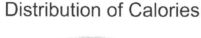

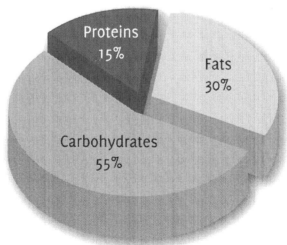

Food Composition Basics—Micronutrients

We have covered the three macronutrients, carbohydrates, fats, and protein. Our diets should also include **micronutrients,** which are substances the body cannot produce by itself but are essential for specific functions. You must include these nutrients in your diet through food and drink. Examples of micronutrients are:

- *Vitamins* including fat-soluble vitamins (A, D, E, K) and water-soluble vitamins (eight B vitamins plus vitamin C).

- *Minerals* (sodium, potassium, chlorine, calcium, phosphorus, magnesium)

- *Trace elements and micro minerals* (zinc, iron, copper, iodine, manganese, selenium, chromium, molybdenum, fluoride, cobalt)

Over the Teeth, Past the Gums, Look Out Stomach, Here It Comes!

Most of the time, we eat without even thinking about what happens after the food passes our lips. But everyone's body is different. Foods that you eat every day may be actually causing your tummy troubles! (We will get to those in Chapter 4.) Please read this chapter first; it will

> One way to take control of your diarrhea is to determine which part of your digestive system is malfunctioning, and then figure out how to correct the problem.

make more sense when we discuss abnormal digestion in later chapters.

Digestion—What Is It?

Digestion is the mechanical and chemical breakdown of food into simpler forms. Your body cannot use the proteins, carbohydrates, or fats directly from the food you eat. It takes a coordinated effort from many systems to make that food usable to the body. First, your food must be broken down into simple building blocks that the body can use for a multitude of functions, such as breathing, contracting muscles, and thinking.

Did you know that digestion actually begins before you even put that first morsel in your mouth? Just the sight, smell, or thought of food initiates a cascade of events that begins in your brain. The brain signals the stomach to start contracting and making gastric juices, all to prepare your body to receive the food.

As we set off on our journey through digestion, you may want to refer to the illustration of the digestive system on the following page.

> The liver, although not directly connected to the stomach or intestines, is a very important organ. It performs over 500 functions.

Mouth to Esophagus

As soon as food enters your mouth, the teeth initiate mechanical breakdown by chewing. The **enzymes** in your saliva chemically digest the simple sugars. Your mouth combines the food and saliva together into a soft gooey ball called a **bolus**.

Digestive System

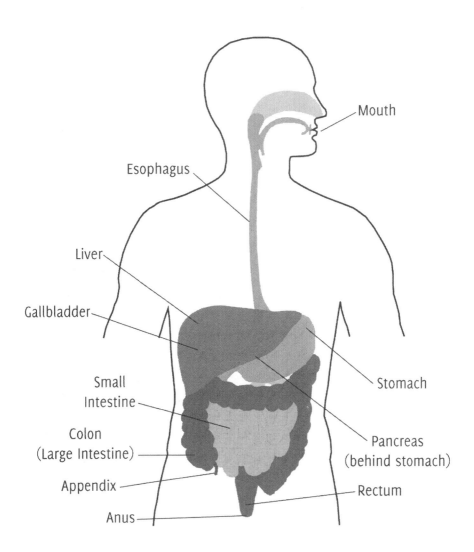

Mouth

Esophagus

Liver

Gallbladder

Small Intestine

Colon (Large Intestine)

Appendix

Anus

Stomach

Pancreas (behind stomach)

Rectum

Esophagus to Stomach

Swallowing takes a coordinated effort from your mouth, tongue, pharynx, and esophagus. The food bolus passes through the **esophageal sphincter**, a valve that allows food into the stomach.

Stomach

The stomach is a flexible, J-shaped organ on the left side of your abdominal cavity (the liver takes up most of the right side). It has four main functions:

- Provides a holding reservoir—it can expand to hold two to four liters of food.

- Grinds the food into smaller particles through strong muscular movements, called **peristalsis**.

- **Denatures** or begins to break down some protein.

- **Secretes** hydrochloric acid to kill almost all the bacteria in your food, while secreting mucus to protect the lining of the stomach from being burned by the acid. When the acid is released, it also signals the pancreas to produce enzymes. These enzymes will soon be needed to digest your food in the small intestine.

> One other important function occurs in the lower portion of the stomach: a **glycoprotein** called **intrinsic factor** is produced. Intrinsic factor must bind with the Vitamin B_{12} in your food so that it can be absorbed in the ileum. (Chapter 17)

Stomach to Small Intestine

Once the food enters the stomach, it takes about two to four hours to mix. The semi-liquid food, now called **chyme**, leaves the stomach through the **pyloric sphincter** and enters the small intestine. The pyloric sphincter regulates how quickly or slowly the chyme leaves the stomach.

28

The timing depends on the size of the meal, how much liquid was consumed, and how much fat and fiber was in the food. Certain conditions (e.g.

> Liquids and simple carbohydrates leave the stomach first, then protein, and lastly, fiber and fat.

gastroparesis, elevated blood sugars) and medications (e.g. narcotic pain relievers) can slow down stomach emptying. Metoclopramide is a medication that speeds up the emptying process.

The small intestine is 20-25 feet (370-462 cm) long, one inch (2.5 cm) in diameter, and consists of three segments:

- **duodenum** (10-12 inches or 15-18 cm in length)
- **jejunum** (8 feet or 148 cm)
- **ileum** (11-12 feet or 203-222 cm)

Duodenum

As the chyme leaves the stomach, it enters the **duodenum**, where iron and calcium are absorbed. The liquid food passes by a small opening, or duct through which bile from the gallbladder and enzymes from the pancreas arrive in the small intestine.

- Bile is produced in the liver and stored in the gallbladder. When foods containing fat need to be digested, the gallbladder releases bile through the common bile duct into the small intestine.
- Pancreatic enzymes are produced in the pancreas and then released through the pancreatic duct into the small intestine.

The bile and pancreatic enzymes break down the carbohydrates, fats, and proteins from long chains into smaller segments. These small building blocks can then be absorbed in the jejunum, the middle section of the small intestine.

Jejunum

The **jejunum** is very important to the digestive process. In the jejunum, carbohydrates, fats and proteins in chyme are simplified into shorter segments that can be absorbed into the bloodstream.

- Simple and complex carbohydrates become glucose
- Fats become fatty acids, which are not absorbed until the ileum
- Proteins become amino acids and peptides

Glucose, fatty acids, amino acids, and peptides are **actively transported** through the cell wall into the bloodstream, where they are delivered to the liver and other organs to be processed into a form that is usable to the body.

Ileum

Nutrients not absorbed in the jejunum continue through to the **ileum**, the final section of the small intestine. The ileum has several unique features:

- Fats, fat-soluble vitamins, Vitamin $B_{12,}$ and magnesium are absorbed
- Bile salts that were released higher in the digestive tract are now "recycled" back into the system

- Fluids and electrolytes are reabsorbed
- It contains immune system cells not found in the duodenum or jejunum

Small Intestine to Large Intestine

The remaining undigested food particles, fiber, and liquid chyme leave the ileum through the ileocecal valve into the cecum. This is the first portion of the **colon**, also called the **large intestine**.

> The ileocecal valve prevents backflow of bacteria from the colon into the small bowel, a condition called **small intestinal bacterial overgrowth (SIBO)**. This topic will be covered in Chapter 16.

The colon begins on your right side, goes straight up (ascending colon), then across the middle of your abdomen (transverse colon), and finally down your left side (descending colon). The colon forms a three-sided frame with the small intestine in the middle. The colon is approximately five feet (150 cm) long and three inches (7.6 cm) in diameter.

The main function of the colon is to absorb water, sodium, and fat-soluble vitamins before the waste leaves the body. In addition, bacteria in the colon ferment, or

> Roughly a liter of liquid stool enters the colon every day. Nearly 99% of the water is reabsorbed before the stool leaves the body.

break down, certain starches, fibers, and sugar alcohols which were not digested by enzymes in the small intestine. (We will discuss these fermentable carbohydrates, also called FODMAPs, in Chapters 4 and 10.) Once broken down, these carbohydrates can be absorbed, providing an additional calorie source in your diet. Byproducts of this fermentation process include hydrogen, methane, and carbon dioxide gases.

As the liquid chyme moves through the large intestine, it gradually becomes more solid as water is reabsorbed back into the body. Finally, the solid waste (called stool) moves through the S-shaped sigmoid colon into the rectum.

Colon to Rectum

When the solid stool arrives in the rectum, it signals the brain that you are ready to have a bowel movement. Coordinated muscles then move the stool through the anus and out of the body.

> Stool is made up of indigestible fiber, bacteria and water.

Transit time is the amount of time it takes for your food to go from mouth to anus. For those with quick transit time (diarrhea), malabsorption of nutrients is a concern. Slowing down the digestion process may provide more time for your body to break down and absorb key nutrients.

> **Myth:**
> Everyone should have a perfectly-formed bowel movement once a day.
>
> **Fact:**
> There is a wide range of "normal" for bowel movements. Transit time varies from a few hours to as long as a week or more. The average time is 18-24 hours.

The Bottom Line

The digestive system is a sophisticated operation with a delicate balance. There are many places where things can get out of sync and cause problems, resulting in diarrhea or its opposite, constipation.

Chapter 3

What is Diarrhea?

Defining Diarrhea

Did you know that there are criteria to define diarrhea? When you have it, you don't care how it's defined. You just want it to go away! Even in the medical community, it has been difficult to attain a consensus for the definition of diarrhea.

Chronic diarrhea is defined by the American Gastroenterological Association as "the production of loose stools with or without increased frequency for more than four weeks."[1] Other medical definitions use frequency of bowel movements in a 24-hour period or measure the volume or weight of the stool.

Am I alone?

"The prevalence of chronic diarrhea in the general population has not been well established... based on a commonly used definition, a reasonable approximation is that chronic diarrhea affects approximately five percent of the population."[2]

Types of Diarrhea

Did you know that all diarrhea is not alike? Depending on the source, there can be between three and five major types. To make it even more confusing, it is possible to have more than one type of diarrhea at a time.

Osmotic Diarrhea

Osmotic diarrhea occurs when the GI tract senses that it is not at a desired state of equilibrium. If certain carbohydrates such as lactose or fructose are not digested properly, the concentration of molecules will be higher inside than outside the intestine. This triggers the bowel to pull extra water into the intestinal tract to balance out the levels, causing very painful cramping and diarrhea.

Osmotic Diarrhea can be found in people who have:

- **Celiac disease** or non-celiac gluten sensitivity
- **Pancreatic insufficiency**
- Carbohydrate intolerance (lactose or fructose)
- Excess consumption of magnesium-containing supplements and medications

With osmotic diarrhea, the output is roughly proportional to the intake of food or liquid. There is one way to tell if

> Making changes to your diet can significantly decrease osmotic diarrhea.

the diarrhea is due to an osmotic process: if you stop eating and drinking, the diarrhea stops.

Inflammatory or Infectious Diarrhea

In inflammatory or infectious diarrhea, the lining of the small intestine may become damaged, so the gut actually "weeps" or oozes. The body not only loses fluid, blood, and other essential nutrients, it also passively loses fluids containing important proteins. This often results in unintentional weight loss. To compound this condition, the damaged intestine may be more sensitive to hyperosmolar foods and beverages, which will be discussed in the next chapter.

Inflammatory or infectious diarrhea can be found in people who have:

- **Inflammatory bowel disease** such as Crohn's disease and ulcerative colitis
- Ischemic colitis
- Colon cancer
- Lymphoma
- Undergone certain types of chemotherapy
- Radiation-induced diarrhea

Inflammatory or infectious diarrhea is less-influenced by diet modifications than osmotic diarrhea.

Dysmotility-Related Diarrhea (Rapid Transit of Stool)

When the nerve impulses and muscular contractions in the gut are not synchronized, food passes through the small intestine too quickly for nutrients and water to be properly absorbed. Medically speaking, this type of diarrhea results from alterations in mechanical stretch receptors.

Dysmotility-related diarrhea can be found in people who have:

- **Irritable bowel syndrome**
- **Carcinoid syndrome**
- Scleroderma
- Undergone full or partial stomach removal (**gastrectomy**)
- Undergone removal (resection) of the colon

- Taken medications that affect peristalsis
- Diabetic neuropathy
- Untreated hyperthyroidism

How, what, and when you eat and drink can alter the speed of food through the digestive system, decreasing chronic dysmotility diarrhea.

Malabsorptive Diarrhea

In malabsorptive diarrhea, the intestinal wall may be compromised. Key macronutrients—carbohydrate, fat, or protein—or micronutrients such as vitamins and minerals are unable to be properly absorbed.

Malabsorptive diarrhea can be found in people with:

- **Steatorrhea** (fat malabsorption diarrhea)
- **Pancreatic insufficiency**
- **Celiac disease**
- **Lactose intolerance**
- History of small bowel resections

Altering your diet can decrease some types of malabsorptive diarrhea, such as lactose intolerance. However, if malabsorption is due to a damaged digestive tract as with celiac disease, diarrhea will likely continue until the intestinal absorptive surface is healed.

Secretory Diarrhea

In secretory diarrhea, the intestinal tract is stimulated to produce high-volume, watery diarrhea, over one liter (4.25 cups) per day. This type of diarrhea causes additional excretion of sodium, chloride, and water, quickly leading to extreme dehydration and, in severe cases, even death. There is no structural damage to the **mucosa**, or lining, of the intestine. However, nutrients may be malabsorbed.

> In some cases of cholera, diarrhea output can exceed one half to one liter per hour.

Secretory Diarrhea can be found in people who have:

- **Carcinoid syndrome**
- VIPoma tumors
- Recently received chemotherapy treatment
- Cholera
- E. Coli
- **Clostridium difficile**

Unfortunately, secretory diarrhea continues even after you stop eating and drinking. Therefore, dietary changes are less effective in controlling this type of diarrhea.

Mechanisms of Diarrhea

Regardless of the cause, there are two primary mechanisms of diarrhea:

- Increased secretion of fluid and electrolytes (e.g. osmotic or secretory diarrhea)
- Decreased absorption of fluid and electrolytes (e.g. inflammatory, infectious, dysmotility, or malabsorptive diarrhea)

Potential Causes of Diarrhea

The following provides a fairly complete list of causes of chronic diarrhea. Most of these diseases and disorders will be addressed in later chapters of this book.

Potential Causes of Diarrhea

- Inflammatory bowel diseases such as Crohn's disease and ulcerative colitis

- Microscopic colitis and various other subtypes of colitis

- Celiac disease

- Irritable bowel syndrome

- Food allergies and sensitivities

- Food intolerances such as lactose or fructose intolerance

- Malabsorption of fat, from diseases such as cystic fibrosis, pancreatic insufficiency, pancreatitis, or pancreatic tumors

- Cancer of the large intestine (colon cancer), or small intestine (adenocarcinoma, lymphoma, carcinoid tumors, or sarcomas)

- Partial blockage of the intestine from hard stool or tumors that allow only liquid stool to pass through

- Endocrine disorders such as hyperthyroidism, diabetes, and Addison's disease

- Bile salt diarrhea

- Small intestinal bacterial overgrowth (SIBO)

- Infection with viruses, bacteria, or parasites

- Chronic alcohol ingestion or abuse

- Surgical resections of major portions of the stomach, small bowel, large bowel, or pancreas

- Eosinophilic gastroenteritis

- HIV and AIDS

- Medications

- Chemotherapy or radiation therapy

- Laxative abuse

- Competitive (especially long distance) running

- Stress

Bristol Stool Chart

The Bristol Stool Chart was created by Dr. Stephen Lewis and Dr. Ken Heaton to analyze and categorize bowel movements.[66] Types one and two are considered constipation, types three and four are "normal" or "desirable" because they pass easily, and types five through seven are different forms of diarrhea.

Bristol Stool Chart

Type 1		Separate hard lumps, like nuts
Type 2		Sausage-shaped but lumpy
Type 3		Like a sausage or snake, but with cracks on its surface
Type 4		Like a sausage or snake, smooth and soft
Type 5		Soft blobs with clear-cut edges
Type 6		Fluffy pieces with ragged edges, mushy
Type 7		Watery, no solid pieces

Bristol Stool Chart used with permission from Dr. SJ Lewis

Stool Color Guide

Your bowel movements can vary quite a bit in color, though anything in the brown tones is considered normal. Food and medications can change the color of your stool.

Red stools can be caused by eating something red, such as a Popsicle, licorice, or beets. Red-colored stools can also result from bleeding hemorrhoids or something more serious, such as cancer or inflammatory bowel disease. Please consult your physician if red stools last more than a week.

Gray stools may be due to lack of bile or if you are taking anti-diarrheal medications.

Black stools may result from eating bananas or black licorice, or taking iron supplements or bismuth subsalicylate (Pepto Bismol®). On the other hand, if there is bleeding in the stomach or high in the digestive tract, the stools may appear black by the time they leave the body. If you have black or "tarry" stools for over a week, please consult your doctor.

While *yellow* stools are normal for breast-fed infants, adults with yellow bowel movements should consult with their doctor. They can indicate fat malabsorption called **steatorrhea**.

Eating green or blue foods or taking multivitamins may lead to *green* bowel movements. Green stools can also be caused by excess bile release from the liver or bile not being stored properly in the gallbladder.

Orange stools can be caused by consuming higher than normal doses of beta-carotene, a pigment in food which is also a precursor to Vitamin A in the body.

The Bottom Line

You may not want to talk about diarrhea, much less analyze it to figure out what type you have. Nevertheless, this information can be very valuable in figuring out what foods you can and can't eat.

Chapter 4

Troublesome Foods, Ingredients, and Intolerances

Up to this point, we have reviewed a lot of technical medical information. This chapter addresses typical dietary causes of diarrhea.

Lactose Intolerance

Lactose intolerance is a common cause of chronic abdominal pain, gas, bloating, and diarrhea. What is **lactose intolerance?** First we need to learn some key terms. **Lactase** is an enzyme that breaks down **lactose**, a type of sugar found in milk. Lactase is produced in the **brush border** of the intestinal **villi** in the first section of the small intestine. When you eat or drink a milk product, the lactose should meet up with the lactase enzymes produced by your body. The lactase helps **hydrolyze**, or break down, the lactose so it can be absorbed. Lactose intolerance occurs when the body does not make enough lactase enzymes to digest lactose. This is called lactase deficiency; there are three primary types.

Types of Lactase Deficiency

- Primary—Referred to as lactose maldigestion, where the activity of the lactase enzyme gradually decreases after weaning. This usually occurs between ages two and twenty and is the most common cause of lactase deficiency in adults. Lactose intolerance may be more common in certain ethnic groups.

- Secondary—Caused by another disorder, such as celiac disease or Crohn's disease, or occurs after bariatric surgery or chemotherapy treatment. Many times, once the initiating disease has been treated and the malabsorption corrected, the ability to produce lactase (and thus digest lactose) returns.

- Congenital—Infants are born with very low or nonexistent levels of intestinal lactase, usually discovered shortly after birth. These babies cannot tolerate breast milk or cow's milk and must be treated with a special lactose-free infant formula. Treatment is a lifelong lactose-free diet.

If you have lactose deficiency and you drink a glass of milk, the lactose is not properly broken down in your small intestine and is still intact when it gets to your colon. Bacteria in your colon are overpowered trying to ferment the excess sugar, which causes gas, bloating, and pain. Meanwhile, the intestine senses the concentrated sugar in the colon and draws in extra water from cells outside the intestine in an attempt to dilute it. This results in osmotic diarrhea, discussed in the previous chapter.

How Is Lactose Intolerance Diagnosed?

A **hydrogen breath test** is the preferred method to diagnose lactose intolerance. This test is administered at a hospital or clinic. Prior to the test, the patient must avoid antibiotics and certain medications for a week or more. In addition, there is a specific diet to follow the day before the test.

After an eight to twelve-hour fast, a breath sample is taken to measure baseline levels of hydrogen. Then 20-25 grams of pure lactose are consumed. Breath readings are then taken at specific intervals for two to three hours. If the level of hydrogen rises higher than 20 ppm (parts per million) between samples, the test is considered positive for lactose malabsorption.

Here in Portland, Oregon, they hydrogen breath test can only be conducted in the Pediatric Gastroenterology Department at Oregon Health and Science University (OHSU). The test costs around $800 and is covered by few insurance companies.

Lactose Challenge

An alternative approach is the lactose challenge. It is a simple way to evaluate your own ability to tolerate lactose.

- Follow a lactose-free diet for five to seven days. Use Appendix D as a reference. Document your GI symptoms using the Food Journal in Appendix A.
- Then, spend three or four days consuming several lactose-containing foods at meals and snacks (ice cream, cheese, milk, yogurt, etc.). Continue keeping a food journal and note your symptoms each day.

Evaluate the results. Did you feel significantly better with no gas, bloating, or diarrhea on the lactose free days? Did you feel awful on the high-lactose days? If so, you may be lactose intolerant.

Remember, it is not always clear-cut for everyone. Lactose intolerance can be a secondary result of a separate undiagnosed problem, such as celiac disease, Crohn's disease, or ulcerative colitis.

If I Have Lactose Intolerance, What Can Be Done About It?

If you have lactose intolerance you have several options. One option, of course, is to completely avoid dairy products. However, that may not be realistic, practical, or even healthy.

Another option is to determine your particular tolerance level through trial and error. Many people with mild lactose intolerance can consume small amounts of lactose without problems, up to two cups spread throughout the day, with no more than four ounces (120 ml) at a time. Keep in mind some people are extremely sensitive; they just *look* at milk and get diarrhea! Good news, research indicates that people can improve their tolerance to lactose by slowly increasing their daily consumption over time.

There are numerous lactose-free options on the market, including lactose-free yogurt, ice cream, cottage cheese, milk, soy milk, rice milk, soy cheese, soy yogurt, and vegan cheese. Find what works best for you, but remember that if you decide to avoid milk products long-term, you will need to take calcium and Vitamin D supplements, as dairy substitutes usually contain less of these important nutrients.

Milk products contain different quantities of lactose. Many people with lactose intolerance can eat yogurt without any problems because the active cultures (*Lactobacillus acidophilus*) help digest the lactose within the yogurt. The dairy products causing the most digestive symptoms tend to be ice cream and milk, while others such as cream, cream cheese, and butter contain little or no lactose and can be consumed without problems. Hard cheeses such as cheddar, Swiss, Colby and Parmesan tend to be better-tolerated than soft cheeses. Interestingly, many people with mild lactose intolerance are able to drink goat's milk, even though it still contains lactose.

The following table summarizes the nutrient information for the common sources of milk.

Nutrient Information for Common Sources of Milk

Type of Milk or Milk Substitute	Calories	Protein (gm)	Fat (gm)	Calcium (mg)	Vit D (IU)	Lactose (grams)
Cow (skim/nonfat)	86	8.4	0.4	299	115	12.5
Cow (whole)	149	7.7	8	276	124	12.3
Lactaid® (calcium enriched, fat free)	90	8	0	500	100	none
Goat	168	8.7	10	327	124	10.4
Soy milk (with added calcium, Vit D)	73	5.8	2	299	114	none
Rice drink	113	0.7	2.3	283	101	none
Almond milk (plain)	90	6	3.5	450	120	none
Hemp milk (Hemp Bliss Original)	110	5	7	20	none	none

Lactase Enzymes

If you have lactose intolerance, I recommend taking Lactaid® or generic-brand lactase enzymes when you eat lactose-containing foods. They merely replace the enzymes your body is lacking. The key is to take them properly and in adequate amounts. Sometimes my patients do not think lactase enzymes help with bloating, gas, and diarrhea. Often they are not taking enough tablets, or are taking them at the wrong time.

Lactaid® caplets come in three forms:

- Fast acting chewable
- Fast acting caplets
- Original strength (three of these equal one fast-acting caplet or chewable!)

I suggest taking one fast-acting Lactaid® tablet with the first bite of food. Then, take another tablet in the middle of the meal to ensure that the enzymes and food are in the intestine at the same time. If you take them 10 minutes before or after the meal, they will not work as effectively.

If you still have digestive symptoms, the next time you consume the same food or drink, increase the dose to two tablets with the first bite of food, and one or two tablets in the middle of the meal. Continue to increase or decrease your dose of Lactaid® until you find the right number of tablets for that particular food.

Personal Story:

I became lactose intolerant at about age 12. For the first few years, I had to avoid dairy products, because Lactaid® tablets were not yet available on the market. Once Lactaid® became available, I quickly learned how many tablets I needed for a particular food to avoid having diarrhea. Back in those days, they only had regular-strength tablets. If I wanted to eat one serving of ice cream, I had to take five or six tablets! Eventually, Lactaid Ultra®, a much stronger version, became available over-the-counter. By age 25, I had my personalized dosing down to a science: two tablets for a piece of cheese, three tablets for cottage cheese, and three or four for a small bowl of ice cream. Thankfully, today's Lactaid® now requires even fewer tablets to treat lactose intolerance.

Fructose Malabsorption

Another potential cause of diarrhea is **dietary fructose intolerance**, also called **fructose malabsorption** (FM).

What is Fructose?

Fructose is a sugar primarily found in fruits, fruit juices, honey, and high-fructose corn syrup; it is also bound to glucose to form sucrose (table sugar).

What is Fructose Malabsorption?

When fructose is consumed, it is absorbed directly into the bloodstream. Fructose malabsorption occurs when fructose from food and drinks is not fully-absorbed in the small intestine. Similar to lactose intolerance, when undigested fructose passes through to the large intestine, it provides food for the colonic bacteria, causing abdominal gas, bloating, pain, and diarrhea.

> Fructose Malabsorption should not be confused with *Hereditary Fructose Intolerance*, a rare genetic disorder which can lead to liver or kidney damage if improperly treated.

Scientists in Australia studying functional gut disorders such as IBS noted that ingestion of fermentable carbohydrates, including fructose and lactose, causes gastrointestinal distress. As a result of these studies, a new dietary treatment has emerged in recent years. It is called the **FODMAP** diet, an acronym for a group of dietary components you probably know little about: Fermentable **O**ligo-, **D**i-, **M**ono-saccharides, **A**nd **P**olyols.

> If you enjoy medical reading, here's an interesting article on FM[34].
> http://www.medicine.virginia.edu/clinical/departments/medicine/divisions/d igestive-health/nutrition-support-team/nutrition-articles/BarrettArticle.pdf

How is FM Diagnosed and Treated?

Similar to lactose intolerance, the best test for FM is the hydrogen breath test. After obtaining a baseline breath sample, 20-25 grams of fructose are consumed. Additional breath samples are taken at specified intervals for two to three hours. Fructose malabsorption is confirmed if hydrogen levels are 20 ppm (parts per million) higher than the lowest previous reading, and are accompanied by gastrointestinal symptoms 30 to 180 minutes after consuming the fructose.

However, as with lactose intolerance, the hydrogen breath test is fairly expensive and not widely available.

Trying out the FODMAP elimination diet may be an easier way to determine if fructose is a problem for you. This diet modifies intake of fructose as well as several other fermentable carbohydrates.

Interestingly, everyone has a different capacity for fructose absorption, and it is quantity-dependent. If you eat a single food containing fructose at a meal you might feel fine. On a different day, you might eat two or three high-fructose foods at one meal, causing uncomfortable digestive symptoms. This may explain why you can tolerate a particular food without problems one day, but another day you eat the same food and feel miserable.

The FODMAP diet will be addressed in more detail in Chapter 10 on irritable bowel syndrome. I recommend the book *IBS—Free at Last!* by Patsy Catsos, MS, RD, LD, as a wonderful guide to embarking on the FODMAP journey.

Fiber

Did you know some types of fiber can worsen diarrhea? In my experience, soluble fiber helps thicken the stools, while insoluble fiber tends to make diarrhea worse for many sufferers. Thus, for my patients, I recommend **increasing soluble fiber** while **limiting insoluble fiber** in the diet.

What Is Fiber?

Fiber is found in the fruits, vegetables, grains, and legumes that we eat. It is the part of the plant that is not digestible by the human body, so it passes through into the stool. Many health experts sing the praises of fiber and its ability to help with both diarrhea and constipation. However, they often forget to discuss the difference between soluble and insoluble fiber.

Neither type of fiber is absorbed into the body, but they affect the intestine in different ways. To make it more complicated, some foods, like nuts, contain both types of fiber. Fruits and vegetables are high in fiber. You can decrease the amount of insoluble fiber by removing the skin, hull, and seeds. One example is an apple—the skin contains insoluble fiber, while the flesh is mainly soluble fiber.

Soluble Fiber

Soluble fiber is fermentable; it attracts water and forms a gel in the digestive system. This chemical process slows down stomach emptying (helping you feel full for longer). Slower digestion can translate into decreased diarrhea.

Foods Containing Soluble Fiber			
flaxseed beans	nuts	potato (no skin)	pears
soybeans	cucumbers	apples	blueberries
dried peas	carrots	psyllium husk	oatmeal
barley	lentils	bananas	oat cereal & oat bran

Health Benefits of Soluble Fiber:

- Decreases stomach emptying. When the stomach empties more slowly, it keeps the blood sugar from rising too quickly. This is helpful for people with hypoglycemia and diabetes.

- Binds to cholesterol in food, leading to decreased total cholesterol and "bad" LDL cholesterol.

Insoluble Fiber

Insoluble fiber, also called cellulose, does not dissolve in water and passes through the body essentially intact. It adds bulk to the stool which is helpful for controlling constipation. Insoluble fiber is often referred to as roughage and is generally found in the plant's husk and peels.

A kernel of wheat consists of three layers:

Diagram of A Wheat Kernel

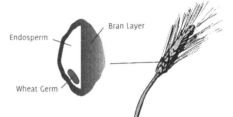

- bran

- endosperm

- germ

The bran, or outermost, layer of wheat contains insoluble fiber, which tends to cause diarrhea.

Foods Containing Insoluble Fiber			
nuts	oats	brown rice	carrots
corn bran (skin)	zucchini	fruit skins (tomato)	celery
cabbage	onions	wheat bran	dried fruit
green beans	whole wheat	dark vegetables	
vegetable skins (potato)		seeds (such as sesame and pumpkin)	

Health Benefits of Insoluble Fiber:

- Decreased risk of diverticular disease and diabetes

- Decreased constipation and hemorrhoids

- Possible decreased risk of colon cancer, although there is conflicting evidence about this

The Low-Fiber Diet in Appendix C limits insoluble fiber but allows soluble fiber. I have highlighted those foods that are considered "thickening" or constipating. Some of these foods are high in soluble fiber, while others have another quality which binds stool together.

How Much Fiber Am I Supposed to Eat Each Day?

Currently, the Institute of Medicine recommends 14 grams of fiber per 1000 calories per day[68]. This generally works out to be a daily intake of about 25-38 grams of total fiber. Studies have shown that most Americans fall quite short of that number, averaging 10-15 grams daily. The guidelines do not specify how much of each type of fiber is recommended.

Let's look at breakfast cereal, for example. The serving size and the amount of fiber per serving vary widely.

Fiber Content of Common Breakfast Cereals

Cereal	Serving Size	Grams of Fiber per serving
Original Fiber One®	½ cup	14 grams
Kashi® GoLean® Crunch	1 cup	8 grams
Kellogg's Raisin Bran®	1 cup	7 grams
General Mills Cheerios®	1 cup	3 grams
Kellogg's Corn Flakes®	1 cup	1 gram

It should be noted that food labels generally list the total grams of fiber, rather than separating out soluble and insoluble. When working toward your daily fiber goal, I suggest you use primarily soluble fiber, which tends to cause less diarrhea.

Polyols or Sugar Alcohols

Polyols, also known as sugar alcohols, are added to products such as sugar-free gum and candy to sweeten the product with fewer absorbed calories. Additionally, they do not contribute to tooth decay or cause sudden increases in blood sugar. This is because polyols are not completely absorbed in the small intestine.

Sugar alcohols cause or exacerbate diarrhea by pulling water into the intestine via osmosis (see Chapter 3). Common types of polyols you will see on an ingredient label include sorbitol, mannitol, xylitol, and erythritol, while less commonly-used ones are maltitol, isomalt, and lactitol.

Everyone has a different tolerance level. Some research indicates that slowly increasing your intake of sugar alcohols daily can result in improved tolerance over time.

Sorbitol

Sorbitol is found naturally in apples, pears, peaches, and prunes. Indeed, prunes and prune juice are extremely effective in the treatment of constipation. Sorbitol is also used commercially in baked goods and baking mixes, jam and jellies, candy, gum, and cough drops. High doses of sorbitol can be prescribed by physicians to treat constipation.

Mannitol

Mannitol is present in celery, onions, pumpkins, strawberries, and mushrooms. Similar to sorbitol, mannitol can be found in commercial candy, jam and jellies, frostings, gum, and cough drops. Some chewable tablets contain mannitol due to its pleasant mouth-feel.

Xylitol

Xylitol is more easily tolerated than sorbitol or mannitol and is less likely to cause gas, bloating, or diarrhea. Xylitol is most commonly used in chewing gum or in liquid medications. It is a very popular choice, because its sweetness and flavor most resembles table sugar.

Erythritol

Erythritol is the newest sugar alcohol and is found in the sweetener Truvia®. Unlike the other polyols, erythritol does not typically cause gastrointestinal distress and is generally well-tolerated. This is because roughly 90 percent is absorbed before it gets to the colon, so it is not fermented by colonic bacteria.

Caffeine

Caffeine is a GI stimulant; it makes everything go through your intestines faster. Simply stated, CAFFEINE CONSUMPTION = MORE DIARRHEA. I find this to be one of the biggest dietary causes of chronic diarrhea in the clients I counsel. Yet, many are reluctant to give up or even decrease their morning caffeine boost.

Caffeine is primarily found in coffee, tea, iced tea, chocolate, colas, and some diet pills. Recent years have seen a boom in the sales of extreme caffeine energy drinks such as Red Bull® and Rockstar®. Another popular source of caffeine is endurance energy supplements such as Clif Shot Bloks® and Jelly Belly Extreme Sport Beans®.

Acidic or Spicy Foods

Eating acidic or spicy foods also speeds up intestinal motility. When you experience diarrhea after consuming these foods, it often burns the skin around the anus, causing pain and itching. Examples of spicy foods to avoid are listed in the miscellaneous section of the Low-Fiber Diet in Appendix C.

> If your bottom is really sore after multiple bouts of diarrhea, try a barrier cream called Calmoseptine®. For more information, you can visit their website:
> http://www.calmoseptineointment.com

Greasy and High-Fat Foods

What do fast food French fries and hamburgers have in common? They are typically high in fat. These types of greasy foods can also cause diarrhea in some individuals.

If we are healthy, the body is very efficient at absorbing fat from the food we eat. After eating high-fat or greasy foods, do your bowel movements...

- Float on top or look oily in the toilet water?
- Have a peculiar odor?
- Seem very light or yellow in color?

If you answered yes to any of these questions, you might have **steatorrhea**. Steatorrhea is a form of fat malabsorption which is abnormal and unhealthy. Those with steatorrhea may have low levels of essential fatty acids, have problems absorbing fat-soluble vitamins, or have significant weight loss due to malnutrition.

Examples of foods containing or consisting primarily of fat include:

- Vegetable shortening and margarine
- Oils, including canola, olive, vegetable, palm, and coconut
- Nuts and seeds
- Marbled meats and meat with visible fat, such as hamburger, ribs, and organ meats, including liver
- Processed meats, such as lunch meat, sausage, hot dogs, and bacon

- Full-fat dairy products, such as ice cream, whipping cream, cheese, butter, and milk

- Desserts, such as pies, cakes, and cookies

Some people experience steatorrhea after gall bladder removal or with other malabsorptive syndromes. If you think you might have steatorrhea, please contact your doctor or gastroenterologist. It can be also be a symptom of a more serious condition or disease.

Osmolality

The easiest way to describe **osmolality** is to tell you it is a measure of a food or drink's concentration level. I often use the terms "richness" or "sweetness" to describe these foods to my clients. For example, let's take a can of frozen orange juice concentrate. It is high in osmolality. When we add extra water to thin it out to the proper concentration, the osmolality is lowered. This is what our intestines do with very concentrated liquids, only extra water is pulled into the intestine to thin out the liquid to a proper concentration level. Consuming foods and liquids high in osmolality often results in severe cramping and diarrhea.

Foods or drinks that are more concentrated than body fluids are called **hyperosmolar** or **hypertonic**. Remember the type of osmotic diarrhea mentioned in Chapter 3? Hyperosmolar foods and liquids cause osmotic diarrhea. Ideally, to be well-tolerated and normally absorbed, foods and drinks should be **isotonic**, or about the same concentration level as body fluids.

Hypertonic Solution

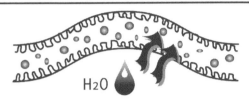

high osmolality food or drink causes
extra water to be pulled into the intestine

Isotonic Solution
(normal absorption)

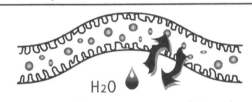

amount of water transported into the
intestine is equal to the amount of water
transported out of the intestine

Osmolality of Common Beverages and Relationship to Serum Osmolality

Liquid/Beverage	Osmolality *mOsm/kg	Relationship to body's osmolality
Normal range of body serum	285-295	--
Oral rehydration solutions	236-397	same
Cow's milk	280-290	same
Gatorade®	297-362	same
Powerade®	346-391	higher
Soda	600-800	higher
Apple juice	339-696	higher

Orange juice	482-612	higher
Grape juice	863	higher
Prune juice	1265	higher
Sherbet	1225	higher
Ice cream	1905	higher
Red wine	2673	higher

*milli-osmoles per kilogram

Since foods and liquids do not come with an osmolality level listed on the nutrition label, you may need to determine your own personal tolerance level. For example, I have discovered that I can eat two pieces of red licorice. However, more than three and I will have diarrhea several hours later. Many of the syrups used in beverages, such as coffees and cocktails (e.g. grenadine, daiquiri mix, liqueurs) are high in osmolality and can exacerbate diarrhea.

Alcohol

Alcoholic drinks stimulate the bowel and worsen diarrhea. In addition, they can be dehydrating. Of all alcoholic drinks, white wine seems to be the best tolerated. The most important advice for alcohol intake? Moderation is best.

Simple Ways to Remember Which Foods Aggravate Diarrhea

Ask yourself...

Is the food:

> Spicy? (horseradish, cayenne)

> Stringy? (celery, cooked spinach)

> Scratchy? (fried or abrasive foods such as bran and granola)

Does it have:

> Skins (most fresh fruits and vegetables)

> Seeds (berries, tomatoes, nuts)

> Sweet syrups (coffee flavorings, high-fructose corn syrup, anything with sugar alcohols)

Will it:

> Swell? (mushrooms)

> Speed up the intestines? (caffeine, alcohol)

The Bottom Line

Figuring out what is causing your diarrhea is challenging. You may find that one, two, all, a combination, or none of these food and beverages increase your trips to the bathroom. There are many ways to tackle the issue of diet and diarrhea. Since you are both the test subject and the control subject, try to isolate as many variables as you can. That way, it is easier to determine if the causes are more related to food, stress, or your environment.

Chart your food intake and bowel movements in a journal (see Appendix A). One method is to choose an elimination diet plan where you remove ALL but a few "safe" (for you) foods for three days. After two or three days, add one new food slowly back into your diet, while journaling your tolerance.

A modified elimination method involves removing only one or two foods for three days at a time. Chart your results. At the end of three days, determine if your diarrhea has lessened. Eliminate the next food(s) for three days, then re-evaluate. Continue this process until all items have been ruled in or out as a cause for your diarrhea. It is very empowering to identify your problem foods. Once this is determined, you have the choice of how much and how often you want to consume a particular food in the future.

Chapter 5

What CAN I Eat?

After discussing which foods might aggravate diarrhea, the invariable question is then asked, "What CAN I eat?" Unfortunately, this simple question does not have an easy answer. Many times I tell my clients, "Eat whatever you tolerate." Admittedly, that isn't very helpful. Let's break down the food groups and see which foods may be easier to digest. Remember, each person tolerates foods differently, so these are general guidelines. If you feel more comfortable with a list of "dos and don'ts," you can refer to the Easy-to-Digest Low-Fiber Diet in Appendix C for a specific listing of foods to choose and avoid.

Carbohydrates and Starches

For the most part, carbs and starches are easy for the body to digest. As discussed in the previous chapter, insoluble fiber is the exception. So initially, I encourage my patients to stick to refined grains, white

> Client tip:
> Many of my patients report eating coconut macaroons helps decrease diarrhea.

rice, pasta, crackers, and breads. It sounds backwards, because much of the healthy nutrition information from the media tells us that we need more whole grains and fiber.

A long-term goal might be to increase your whole grains. However, in the short term, I suggest removing the whole grains and insoluble fiber until your digestive system calms down. When you are feeling better, add small amounts of fiber-containing foods and gradually increase quantities as tolerated.

Meats and Proteins

Choose meat, poultry, and fish that are well-cooked, tender, baked, barbequed, boiled, broiled, and not

> Don't forget to chew your food thoroughly, it helps digestion.

too spicy. Watch out for super-sweet (high osmolality) marinades, soups, and sauces. Creamy peanut butter and other nut butters are generally tolerated, while nuts and seeds are not. Eggs are an excellent source of protein, and most people can eat them without difficulty. Smooth tofu is another good choice.

I generally do not recommend eating beans and legumes initially, as they tend to cause gas and bloating, even in people without digestive problems. As you become more comfortable in knowing how your body responds to particular foods, you may begin to include eat small quantities of canned beans (start with refried) as tolerated.

Many of my clients report that they tolerate meat, poultry, and fish better when it contains fewer chemicals. It is expensive to purchase free-range, grain-fed, and antibiotic-free animal products, but if it results in less diarrhea, the trade-off might be worth it.

Fruits

This is a challenging food group. Most people can eat small amounts of raw fruit without problems. Ripe bananas and avocados are usually well-tolerated. I suggest eating mostly canned fruit without skins and seeds.

> Eating a lot of fruit at one time may worsen diarrhea.

As your diarrhea improves, slowly increase your intake of raw fruit. I would suggest beginning with melons and peeled apples. Some of my patients find that juicing or making smoothies improves their tolerance to fruits and vegetables. This also allows a wider variety of food choices.

Vegetables

As with fruits, choose primarily canned vegetables without skins and seeds. Well-cooked vegetables are also a good option. Try well-cooked green beans, beets, summer squash, zucchini, carrots, yams, or peeled potatoes. From personal and professional experience, corn, popcorn, and lettuce tend to be the most difficult foods to digest.

Dairy

If you tolerate lactose and do not have a dairy protein allergy, you may consume dairy in desired quantities, within the context of a healthy overall diet. Children over age nine and adults need about three servings of milk products per day. What counts as a serving?

- Eight ounces of low-fat or fat-free milk or yogurt
- 1/3 cup shredded cheddar

- Two (¾ oz) slices of Swiss cheese
- ½ cup pudding or frozen yogurt, each counting as a half serving

A word of warning—higher fat dairy products such as heavy cream, half and half, and ice cream may aggravate GI distress. Low-fat yogurt is a good choice; it contains desirable quantities of protein, carbs, and fat, and is an excellent source of calcium and probiotics.

Fats

Some people find that excess fat worsens diarrhea, so choose small to moderate quantities of healthier fats, such as olive oil, canola oil, and nut butters, while decreasing trans and saturated fats. (Chapter 2)

Other Ingredients to Try

There are numerous "natural" treatments for diarrhea; many of these are for acute rather than chronic issues. Listed below are natural ingredients that people have used to treat chronic diarrhea.

Chamomile

Chamomile is a natural pain reliever which reportedly rids your body of cramps and inflammation. It is available in tea, capsule, and liquid form. Chamomile may be effective for those suffering from mild to moderate diarrhea.

Peppermint

Peppermint relaxes the intestinal muscles, reducing cramping, pain, gas, and diarrhea. Peppermint is typically consumed in tea or as oil packaged in enteric-coated capsules. There have been reports of allergies to peppermint. Please consult with your doctor or pharmacist before taking high doses of this plant.

Pectin

Did you know that pectin is an age-old cure for diarrhea as well as constipation? Pectin occurs naturally in fruits such as apples, plums, and oranges. The most common use of pectin is as a thickening agent in making jams and jellies.

As a soluble fiber, it absorbs water and forms a gel that increases the volume of the stool. In 2003, the FDA ruled that scientific evidence does not support the use of pectin for diarrhea. However, many people still treat their diarrhea with pectin capsules.

Spices Reported to Reduce Diarrhea

I cannot speak from personal experience, but some patients have fewer digestive symptoms when they use certain herbs and spices.

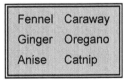

Fennel Caraway
Ginger Oregano
Anise Catnip

The Bottom Line

In practical terms, if you tolerate it, you can eat it. That said, just because you tolerate a particular food does not mean you need to subsist on it. For example, many of my patients tolerate potato chips, so they tend to eat them in large quantities. ("But it's the one food I can eat without getting diarrhea!") This does not mean you should eat *only* chips!

Remember, the goal is to consume an overall healthy diet—think moderation and variety—with the understanding that you may not be able to tolerate certain foods at certain times.

Chapter 6

Constipation and Constipating Foods

If you are reading this book because you have chronic diarrhea, you might think that chronic constipation would be preferable. Let me assure you, those who have this condition face many challenges as well.

Many people with IBS or functional bowel disorders often have alternating diarrhea and constipation. It can be frustrating to be eating one way for diarrhea, then have to switch it all around when they become constipated.

Just as some foods can cause diarrhea, the following foods may thicken stool, which is great for diarrhea but can worsen constipation. If you are familiar with the antiquated **BRAT** diet, then these foods may be familiar to you. The **BRAT** diet consists of **B**ananas **R**ice **A**pplesauce and **T**oast. Sometimes you may see an extra **T** on the end of **BRATT** which stands for **T**ea, or **BRATTY** with **Y** for **Y**ogurt.

Constipating Foods

- Fruits: bananas, applesauce
- Breads and starches: oatmeal, rice, pasta, potatoes, pretzels
- Proteins: peanut butter, cheese (especially cheddar)
- Miscellaneous: gelatin, boiled milk, cornmeal (used in foods such as corn chips or corn bread), tapioca, marshmallows, and (some of my patients swear by) coconut macaroons.

(Note: constipating foods are highlighted on the Easy-to-Digest Diet in Appendix C)

Recommendations for Chronic Constipation

The Academy of Nutrition and Dietetics recommends the following strategies for chronic constipation[7]:

- Eat adequate fiber, especially through intake of fruits and vegetables. The goal is to consume five to seven servings of fruits and vegetables daily, gradually increasing to 25 to 38 grams of fiber daily. Fiber sources include psyllium, inulin, and oligosaccharides.

- Increase fluid intake to a minimum of 64 ounces (8 cups or almost two liters) daily. Drink a hot beverage at breakfast to stimulate intestinal motility.

- Participate in daily exercise or physical activity.

- Consider adding bulk-forming agents such as psyllium, calcium polycarbophil, or methylcellulose. (Chapter 9)

- Add pre/probiotics. (Chapter 8)

- Avoid stool retention: heed the urge to use the bathroom about 30-45 minutes after a meal. Consider initiating a bowel retraining program. Examples:

http://www.aboutconstipation.org/site/about-constipation/treatment/bowel-retraining

http://www.med.unc.edu/ibs/files/educational-gi-brochures/BowelRetrain.pdf

Over-the-Counter Remedies or Medications for Constipation

The following remedies are listed from relatively mild to more invasive. Please consult with your doctor or pharmacist before starting any new medication. Remember, just because a medication is available over-the-counter does not mean it is harmless.

- Fruit-Eze™ regularity blend is an all-natural laxative alternative made of prunes, raisins, dates, and prune juice http://fruiteze.com/

- Sorbitol or other sugar alcohol

- Stool softeners (docusate, Colace®, Correctol®)

- Mineral oil

- Milk of magnesia ("MOM")

- Magnesium citrate

- Glycerin suppositories

- Enemas

- Polyethylene glycol or MiraLAX® http://www.miralax.com/miralax/home/index.jspa

The Bottom Line

Some people with chronic diarrhea also suffer from intermittent constipation. Knowing the dietary and medical treatment for both extremes is important. Before starting any new medication or over-the-counter supplements, always discuss them with your doctor and pharmacist.

Chapter 7

The Effects of Stress

Types of Stress

A stressor is anything that causes stress for a person. They tend to fall into five main categories:

- Physical—surgery, trauma
- Psychological—depression, anxiety, grief, anger
- Biological—chronic disease, chronic pain, illness
- Environmental—toxins, pollution, noise
- Sociological—living situation, marriage or relationship problems

The connection between stress and diarrhea is undeniable. For some, stressors trigger diarrhea, while for others, diarrhea *is* the stressor. Many times we believe we have control over physical and environmental types of stressors, but often we feel powerless over biological stressors, such as cancer or chronic disease.

Type A Personality

In my experience, the majority of people with chronic diarrhea are those with what are sometimes called Type A personalities. Do you fit the stereotype?

Driven	Confident	Manager
Detail-oriented	Ambitious	Multi-tasking
Controlling	Outgoing	Impatient
Competitive	High-strung	Work-a-holic

Often these people fall victim to various physical maladies. These can include chronic headaches, back pain, insomnia, and yes, diarrhea. (I put myself in this category!)

Caretaker Personality

Another type of person I see with chronic diarrhea is one described with a "caretaker" or "people pleaser" personality. These people are concerned with the wants and needs of others, often putting these needs ahead of their own. Over time, we tend to see what years of caretaking can do—the caretaker's health has been compromised as a result.

Stress Relief

There are many effective strategies to alleviate stress. Some find relief in prayer, yoga, meditation, relaxation therapy, hypnosis, biofeedback, or exercise. Others find it through massage therapy or acupuncture. I encourage you to find whatever method works for you! An interesting article titled, "Behavioral Therapy for IBS" can be found at: www.webmd.com/ibs/guide/behavioral-therapy

Scientists are studying the effects of Corticotropin-releasing factor (CRF), which may play a key role with stress and IBS. In the future, we may have medications that target CRF to control IBS.

Can Subconscious Stress Cause Diarrhea?

In the late 1990's I read a fascinating book called *The Mindbody Prescription* by Dr. John Sarno. Dr. Sarno conducted his own research and reached conclusions from those studies. Unfortunately, his studies were not double-blind, **randomized, controlled trials (RCT)**, which form the foundation of medical science. However, my years of professional and personal experience have demonstrated how his theories can apply in real life.

Dr. Sarno describes how people with Type A and caretaker personalities can have excessive stress in their subconscious minds. When their subconscious is overflowing with stress—Dr. Sarno calls it rage—the body shunts oxygen to certain parts of the body, resulting in pain. This pain manifests itself differently in each individual, causing migraine headaches in one person, carpal tunnel in someone else, and back pain in yet another. I theorize that diarrhea can be another manifestation of this problem. Dr. Sarno recommends bringing these stressors from the subconscious to the conscious mind, where they can be dealt with on a conscious level. You address your own stressors through daily journaling, essay writing, and positive verbalization, telling yourself, "No, brain, I am not going to let you cause that pain/diarrhea today. I am going to deal with this stress directly."

In the book, he also notes that if the root cause of the stress is not addressed, the pain might shift from one area of the body to another. Dr. Sarno's research may sound far-fetched, but I have personally experienced improvement of my pain through his techniques.

Furthermore, I have seen positive results in my clients. I encourage you to work through the stressors in your life and see the effect it has on your diarrhea.

The Bottom Line

No one is immune to stress. We can all find better ways to cope with the pressures in our lives. Finding better ways to manage stress can relieve pain and diarrhea as well!

Chapter 8

Probiotics and Prebiotics

For over a decade, I have recommended a trial of probiotics to virtually all of my patients. Why? Of all the strategies I discuss with clients, adding probiotics has resulted in the most significant decrease in chronic diarrhea. Want to know if you need probiotics? Read on.

What Are Probiotics?

Probiotics are a vast group of living microbial organisms comprising normal gastrointestinal flora. Put simply,

> The average human intestine contains **over 400 types of probiotic bacteria!**

probiotics are *good bacteria* that are *supposed* to live in your intestinal tract. They protect you, the host, while preventing disease. An imbalanced bacterial population in your gut is also known as **dysbiosis.**

Examples of probiotics include bacterial species *Lactobacillus and Bifidobacterium*, as well as the *Saccharomyces* yeasts. In 1965, researchers coined the term "probiotics," though the concept and use of beneficial bacteria to promote health had been around since the early 1900s.

Scientists have agreed on four benefits of probiotics, despite not knowing their exact mechanisms[15]:

- Suppress growth and prevent "bad" (disease-causing) bacteria from adhering to intestinal walls

- Maintain and stimulate the healthy cells of the intestinal lining to optimize immune function
- Enhance functioning of the immune system
- Modulate perception of pain

Other possible benefits of using probiotics:

- Signal cells to strengthen mucus in the intestine, providing a barrier against infection
- Destroy the toxins released by "bad" bacteria

What Are Prebiotics?

Prebiotics are *nondigestible fibers and complex sugars* that promote the growth and metabolic activity of the beneficial bacteria, primarily the *Bifidobacterium,* in the colon. They provide fuel for the probiotics already living in the intestine, favoring the good bacteria over the harmful ones. A prebiotic *may* be a fiber, but not all fibers are prebiotic.

Prebiotics were not defined until 1995. One example of a prebiotic is inulin, found in Jerusalem artichokes and asparagus stems. Fructooligosaccharides (FOS), which occur naturally in garlic, onions, green bananas, zucchini, watermelon, and peaches, are another type of prebiotic.

Health benefits of taking prebiotics:

- Possibly lowers cholesterol
- Increases stool weight
- Decreases transit time

- Increases calcium absorption
- Increases *Bifidobacterium* in the colon

Many reputable health resources recommend taking both prebiotics and probiotics. However, it is my experience that those who suffer from IBS-D (diarrhea predominant) or who are FODMAP-sensitive do not tolerate prebiotics; it exacerbates their diarrhea. (Chapter 10)

Synbiotics and Functional Foods

Fermented milk products such as yogurt and kefir are considered **synbiotic** because they contain both the live probiotic bacteria and the prebiotic fuel working synergistically. Products containing prebiotics, probiotics, or both are also called **functional foods**.

Functional foods exert a potentially positive effect on health beyond basic nutrition. One example is yogurt. Beyond the benefits of carbohydrate, protein, fat, and calcium contained in the yogurt itself, it contains active cultures of *L. acidophilus*, providing additional health benefits via probiotics. Functional food products containing prebiotics and/or probiotics include cereals, bread, beverages, yogurt, and nutritional supplements.

History of Probiotic Use

For thousands of years, the food we ate was unrefrigerated, unpasteurized, and unprocessed. Over the past hundred-plus years, the U.S. has improved food processing to prevent harmful bacteria and toxins from entering our food supply. While this has prevented many types of dangerous illnesses, it has resulted in fewer beneficial bacteria living in our gut as well.

Why Is It Important to Have Good Bacteria Living in Our Gut?

The intestine is our first line of defense against harmful pathogens, chemicals, and preservatives that we do not want in our bodies. In order to fight these invaders, the cells in the small intestine tightly line up

> Sixty to seventy percent of the body's immune cells are located in the gastrointestinal tract.

next to each other, forming an impermeable barrier. Probiotics assist the cells in maintaining these **tight junctions**.

One leading scientific hypothesis proposes that dysbiosis allows tight junctions to loosen up, resulting in **leaky gut syndrome** or **intestinal permeability**. Openings created between the cells may permit proteins or toxins cross the intestinal barrier. Once the foreign invaders are inside, **antibodies** are created as the immune system is activated. Many autoimmune and gastrointestinal disorders have been linked to leaky gut syndrome; these include Crohn's disease, celiac disease, Type 1 diabetes, psoriasis, and eczema.

Leaky Gut Syndrome
(Intestinal Permeability)

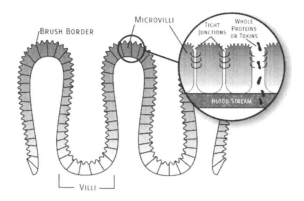

What Makes a Good Probiotic?

To maximize their effectiveness, probiotics must remain stable in the acidity of the stomach and the alkalinity of the duodenum. Further down the GI tract, they must adhere to the surface of the small intestine and effectively populate the colon.

Dietary Sources of Probiotics

The dietary use of live bacteria dates back thousands of years. Yogurt is the most common and familiar form of probiotic, which contains primarily *Bifidobacterium* and *Lactobacillus* species. However, fermented dairy beverages such as kefir actually contain a higher concentration of live cultures. In today's marketplace, you can also find probiotics in soup, cheese, energy bars, even cereal.

There is a downside to getting probiotics exclusively from food sources. It is very difficult to determine how much bacteria are surviving both the stomach acid and bile in order to assert their positive effects.

Probiotic Supplements

If my client is taking probiotics to "promote good gut health," I support exclusive use of food sources of probiotics. However, if a patient is actively experiencing gastrointestinal symptoms from a known disease or disorder, I typically recommend they add an over-the-counter probiotic supplement to their daily regimen.

Probiotic supplements are formulated with a special coating to withstand stomach acid and bile before dissolving in the small intestine. Once the probiotics are released, they can adhere to the intestinal wall and support immune system function.

Probiotic Research

The past decade has seen an increase in the number of scientific studies on the effectiveness of probiotic supplements. However, one difficulty in creating a clinical trial is the wide variety of yeasts and bacteria species available. In scientific studies, many probiotics are used individually or in combination with other bacteria or yeasts. Studies have shown that some species are more effective in treating a particular disorder or disease.

Even more frustrating, not all probiotic supplements are alike. When independent companies test products, they find wide variability in the quantity and potency of live bacteria in each capsule. Many capsules do not even contain the quantity of live bacteria stated on the bottle.

Probiotic Supplement Consistency

ConsumerLab.com, LLC (CL) is an independent testing company. Dietary supplements and herbs are tested for potency; this information is released to help consumers and healthcare professionals determine which products to use or recommend. CL publishes results of its tests at www.consumerlab.com, in its book *ConsumerLab.com's Guide to Buying Vitamins and Supplements*, and in special technical reports[16].

They periodically test different brands of probiotics to evaluate their potency (how many millions of bacteria claimed on the packaging vs. the actual amount of bacteria in each capsule).

Which Probiotic Should I Take and How Much?

It is challenging to provide detailed recommendations on which probiotic supplement to take and what dosage, due to variability in strength and viability. I do not recommend one particular brand over another, primarily because information changes quickly, and specific probiotics may be better-suited for a particular medical condition. The following table presents different conditions and the species of probiotic which has been scientifically studied and proven effective for that particular disease or disorder.

Use of Specific Probiotic Strains in Gastrointestinal Diseases and Disorders

Disease or Disorder	Strain of Probiotic used for targeted treatment
H. Pylori infection	*Lactobacillus casei* Shirota
Lactose Intolerance	*Lactobacillus bulgaricus*
IBS	*Bifidobacterium infantis, Sacchromyces boulardii, Lactobacillus plantarum,* and combination probiotics *Bacillus coagulans* GBI-30, PTA-6086 (marketed as Digestive Advantage®)
Ulcerative colitis	*E. coli* Nissle, and a mixture of several strains of *Lactobacillus, Bifidobacterium* and *Streptococcus* may be most beneficial.
Infectious diarrhea	*Lactobacillus rhamnosus* and *Lactobacillus casei* may be particularly helpful in treating diarrhea caused by rotavirus. Several strains of *Lactobacillus* and a strain of the yeast *Saccharomyces boulardii* may help treat and shorten the course of infectious diarrhea.
Clostridium difficile	*Saccharomyces boulardii*
Antibiotic-associated Diarrhea (AAD)	Various probiotic strains, including *Lactobacillus, Bifidobacterium, Saccharomyces, Streptococcus, Enterococcus,* and/or *Bacillus,* are associated with a decrease in AAD

The International Scientific Association for Probiotics and Prebiotics (ISAPP), in *The P's and Q's of Probiotics: A Consumer Guide for Making Smart Choices,* recommends looking at these four criteria prior to choosing a probiotic[17].

- *Probiotic Strain*

  Try to match the particular strain with published scientific research. This is challenging, but important. Not all products are equal.

- *Proof*

  Probiotics must be tested on humans to determine health benefits. Does the product contain the same quantities as the published studies?

- *Quality and Quantity*

  Probiotics can be effective at varying strengths. Scientific studies have determined health benefits from 50 million to over 1 trillion colony forming units (CFUs) per day. A probiotic with higher CFUs does not necessarily equal better quality or effectiveness.

- *Package*

  What does the package label say? Strain, quantity of CFUs, serving size, health benefits, proper storage conditions, expiration date, and additional corporate contact information should all be included.

After making your choice based on the criteria above, I suggest taking one brand of probiotic for several weeks. (You may be able to obtain free samples by contacting a company directly.) If you do not notice significant improvement in your gas, bloating, or diarrhea after that time, don't up—try a different brand.

Guidelines for taking probiotics:

- Use the dosing recommended on the product label. Generally, dosing is one capsule two to three times per day on an empty stomach. If taking three capsules per day, take the first one right after you wake up, one in the afternoon, and the last one before bed.

- Do not take the probiotic with a hot beverage or cereal, as the heat might destroy some of the good bacteria.

- Try probiotics for at least three to six months. Consider cutting back to one capsule a day after two months and note any changes.

- Eat yogurt (minimum 6-10 ounces per day) or kefir. Remember, not all live cultures in yogurt survive well in the acidic stomach environment.

- If taking prescription antibiotics, *wait two hours before taking the probiotic* so they do not cancel each other out. Remember, antibiotics will kill off both the good *and* bad bacteria. One exception: you may continue to take a yeast probiotic (such as FloraStor®), with your antibiotic. Antibiotics do not interfere with a yeast probiotic.

The following table lists some common name-brand probiotics that have been studied and proven effective in delivering the good bacteria to the intestine.

Brand-Name Probiotics and Their Targeted Treatments

Brand Name	Type of Probiotic	Primary treatment	Website
Align®	-*Bifidobacterium infantis* 35624	-Overall digestive health -IBS	http://www.aligngi.com/
Digestive Advantage®	-*Bacillus coagulans* GBI-30, PTA-6086	-IBS -Lactose intolerance -Constipation	http://digestiveadvantage.com/products.asp
Phillips' Colon Health®	-*Lactobacillus gasseri* KS-13 -*Bifidobacterium bifidum* G9-1 -*Bifidobacterium longum* MM-2	-Occasional constipation -Diarrhea -Gas, bloating	http://colonhealthprobiotic.com/

Culturelle®	-Lactobacillus Rhamnosus GG	-Improved digestive function -Immune support	http://www.culturelle.com/
FloraStor®	-Saccharomyces boulardii lyo	-C. Diff -IBD -HIV/AIDS-associated diarrhea	http://florastor.com/
Mutaflor®	-Escherichia coli Nissle 1917	-Ulcerative colitis -Crohn's disease -Chronic diarrhea -IBS -Pouchitis	http://mutaflor.ca/ *Mutaflor® is no longer available for purchase in the US due the change in classification from "medical food" to "biologic"
VSL #3®	-Bifidobacterium breve -Bifidobacterium longum -Bifidobacterium infantis -Lactobacillus acidophilus -Lactobacillus plantarum -Lactobacillus paracasei -Lactobacillus bulgaricus -Streptococcus thermophilus	-Ulcerative colitis -IBS -Ileal pouchitis	http://www.vsl3.com/

Who *Should NOT* Take a Probiotic?

- People over 65 years old who are in poor health

- Young children

- People with comprised immune systems; especially avoid probiotics containing *Saccharomyces* yeasts

- Possibly those with **Small Intestinal Bacterial Overgrowth** (Chapter 16)

Do Probiotic Supplements Have any Side Effects?

Some people experience gas and bloating when beginning probiotics. It may take two to four weeks for those symptoms to subside while the good bacteria insert themselves into the intestine.

Occasionally, I will have a patient experience more severe symptoms when they first begin taking probiotic supplements. This reaction is sometimes referred to as the Jarisch-Herxheimer (or "Herx") reaction. It occurs when the bad bacteria are dying off and the body is unable to release the toxins quickly enough. In the short-term—days to a few weeks—these toxins can exacerbate the symptoms being treated and cause more gas, bloating, or diarrhea. They may also create their own flu-like symptoms including headache, joint and muscle pain, body aches, sore throat, general malaise, sweating, chills, or nausea.

If you experience the Herx reaction, it is best to cut back on the dosage, while continuing to take probiotics until the toxins are eliminated from the body. Charcoal tablets taken about two hours after the probiotics can help bind and remove the toxins. Please discuss this with your doctor and pharmacist.

Once the harmful bacteria have been eliminated, it is time for the probiotics to do their job.

The Bottom Line

Probiotics are generally well tolerated. Many of my clients notice immediate improvement in their GI symptoms within the first week. The most frequent gastrointestinal complaints while using probiotics are gas and constipation. If no significant improvement is noted in the first month, consider changing brand, dose, or bacteria strain of probiotic.

Chapter 9

Medications and Diarrhea

This chapter will discuss medications: those that can cause diarrhea, those for treatment of diarrhea, and how medications have the potential to be malabsorbed in certain medical conditions. We will also cover bulking agents and fibers, such as Metamucil®.

I am not a doctor or a pharmacist, I am a dietitian. So, while I cannot prescribe medications for the treatment of diarrhea, I do have professional experience with many of my patients taking these medications. In addition, this chapter was reviewed by for accuracy and comprehensiveness by two pharmacists.

Diarrhea as a Side Effect from Medications

Prescribed medications are available for a multitude of maladies and conditions, from high blood pressure and diabetes to anxiety and infection. These medications can restore health and improve quality of life. Unfortunately, diarrhea can be a frequent side effect of both prescribed and over-the-counter (OTC) medications.

When a patient comes to see me for diarrhea, I look carefully at their medication list to see if diarrhea is listed as a common side effect. If the answer is "yes," I recommend they discuss this with their doctor and/or pharmacist. Sometimes other medications in the same class can be substituted, which may lessen diarrhea.

Prescribed and OTC Medications with Diarrhea as a Common Side Effect

Antibiotics (any, but particularly)
Cephalosporins
Clindamycin
Sulfonamides
Erythromycin
Neomycin
Tetracycline
Ampicillin
Amoxicillin
Fluoroquinolones (i.e. Ciprofloxacin)
Any broad-spectrum antibiotic

Antihypertensives and Cardiac Drugs
Reserpine
Guanethidine
Methyldopa
Guanabenz
Guanadrel

Quinidine
Digitalis
Digoxin
Procainamide
Beta-blockers
ACE-inhibitors
Angiotensin II receptor blockers
Diuretics (Acetazolamide, Ethacrynic
    acid, Furosemide)

Neuropsychiatric drugs
Lithium
Fluoxetine
Alprazolam
Valproic acid
Ethosuximide
L–Dopa
Meprobamate

Bile Acids
Chenodeoxycholic acid
Ursodeoxycholic acid

Cholinergics
Metoclopramide
Neostigmine
Bethanechol

Gastrointestinal Drugs
5-aminosalycilates (especially
    Olsalazine)
Antacids (diarrhea increases with
    those containing
    magnesium; those
    containing calcium
    are more constipating)
Milk of magnesia (MOM)
Proton pump inhibitors (Nexium,
    Protonix)
H2-receptor antagonists (Tagamet,
    Zantac)
Misoprostol
Laxatives
Lactulose
Sorbitol

Hypolipidemic agents
Clofibrate
Gemfibrozil
HMG–CoA reductase inhibitors
    (lovastatin, fluvastatin,
    pravastatin)
Cholestyramine

Miscellaneous
Antiparkinsonian drugs (Levodopa)
Oral hypoglycemia agents
    (Metformin)
Thyroid hormones (Synthroid)
Some chemotherapeutic agents
NSAIDs (aspirin, ibuprofen,
    naproxen)
Phenylbutazone
Mefenamic acid
Auranofin
Colchicine
Theophylline
Tacrine
Anticholinergic agents
Vitamin C
Magnesium

Antibiotic-Associated Diarrhea

The past several decades have seen a rise in antibiotic-resistant organisms. While doctors are now more selective when prescribing antibiotics, some illnesses and infections still require this important treatment.

The purpose of antibiotics is to kill the harmful bacteria which cause infection. However, in the process, many of the good bacteria in the gut (Chapter 8) are killed off as well. This can result in what doctors refer to as **antibiotic-associated diarrhea (AAD)**. If the good bacteria are not replaced through the addition of probiotics, diarrhea can continue long-term.

Successful Case Study:

I had a patient who had a colonoscopy two years earlier. During the procedure, the colon was accidentally perforated, which led to an infection. Luckily, he did not require surgical repair. Instead, he was given several antibiotics over the course of the 10-day hospitalization.

Soon after discharge, he began having four to six loose stools daily. By the time he met with me, two years had gone by, and he was tired of having diarrhea. While reviewing his diet, I noticed he did not eat yogurt or consume any foods containing probiotics. I recommended one capsule of probiotic twice a day for six months. He began treatment, and within one week, he happily reported that he was down to one or two normal stools per day.

Clostridium difficile

Some bacterial illnesses require treatment with a broad-spectrum antibiotic, such as clindamycin. These wide coverage antibiotics can alter gut flora or normal bacteria, leaving it susceptible to other harmful bacteria. One of these is **Clostridium difficile**, commonly known as C. diff, a bacterium that can populate the colon and cause massive amounts of diarrhea. If left untreated, C. diff can result in pseudomembranous colitis or a life-threatening condition called toxic megacolon, where the colon rapidly dilates and the body can go into septic shock. Symptoms of C. diff include:

- Severe diarrhea (in excess of five to ten stools per day), with a peculiar, potent odor, different from typical diarrhea
- Fever
- Abdominal pain and/or tenderness
- Rapid heart rate
- Dehydration

How Is Clostridium difficile Diagnosed?

Clostridium difficile is diagnosed with a stool sample. If you have recently been treated with antibiotics and have symptoms of C. diff, contact a physician immediately.

How Is Clostridium difficile Treated?

Standard treatment for C. Diff includes taking a course of antibiotics, either vancomycin or metronidazole. Unfortunately, C. diff commonly recurs. Some studies have shown probiotics such *Saccharomyces boulardii,* a yeast, may be effective in both treating and preventing recurrence of C. diff. However, there are risks associated with introducing yeast to an immune-compromised system, so it is not recommended as part of standard therapy.

New experimental treatments include a preventative vaccine and fecal transplant, which involves transplanting a healthy donor's stool into the patient's body. In a five-minute office procedure, donated feces are inserted into the recipient's rectum with a small injector. Studies with fecal transplant are very promising; it may become the primary treatment for C. diff in years to come.

Take Probiotics with Antibiotics!

Scientific studies suggest it is reasonable to give probiotics to both adults and children who have been prescribed antibiotics. This includes those with presumed infectious diarrhea. In May 2012, the *Journal of the American Medical Association* released a meta-analysis, a study combining and analyzing the results of 82 **randomized controlled trials** on antibiotic-associated diarrhea[18]. The authors concluded that "probiotics are associated with a reduction in antibiotic-associated diarrhea."

When Should I Take Probiotics with My Antibiotics?

Take the probiotics at least two hours after you take your prescribed antibiotic so they do not compete with each other. (Chapter 8)

Medications for Treatment of Diarrhea

There are many over-the-counter and prescription medications available to treat diarrhea. They have different modes of action and side effects; some work better for certain people and conditions.

I was unable to locate a reference in a physician or pharmacy textbook describing the types of medications available for the treatment of diarrhea. With the help of a pharmacist colleague, we created the table on the following pages.

Medications for Treatment of Diarrhea

Type and Generic Name	Brand Name	How it Works	Side Effects	Comments
Adsorbents—nonspecific, adsorbs chemicals, toxins, infectious organisms, nutrients, and digestive juices				
Bismuth Subsalicylate	Pepto-Bismol® Kaopectate®	-Not completely understood, but is thought to coat the intestinal lining -Reduces fluid output (antisecretory)-Reduces intestinal inflammation (anti-inflammatory) -Kills some bacteria that cause diarrhea (antibacterial)	May cause constipation, blackening of tongue or stool	-Should not be used by children with flu or chicken pox due to risk of Reye's Syndrome -Has been shown so decrease traveler's diarrhea -Should not be used with patients on Coumadin
Anti-Motility Agents (Over-the-Counter)				
Loperamide	Imodium® Pepto Diarrhea Control®	-Slows down peristalsis, allows more time for water to be absorbed from stool -Decreases the urge to have a bowel movement after a meal (called the **gastrocolic reflex**)	Dizziness, drowsiness	-Should not use if E. coli, Clostridium difficile, or salmonella is suspected -Does not cross the blood-brain barrier, so does not cause euphoria like some of the opioid medications -Mild opiate withdrawal possible after stopping long-term therapy

Anti-Motility Agents (Prescription Medications)

Codeine Phosphate		-Slows down peristalsis -Provides pain relief	Dizziness, drowsiness, constipation; May be habit-forming	-Occasionally used for IBS-D -Can cause withdrawal symptoms if drug suddenly stopped
Diphenoxylate	Lomotil®	-Slows down peristalsis -Provides pain relief	Crosses the blood-brain barrier and can be habit forming when used long-term in high doses. Can eventually build up a tolerance	-Contains atropine -Cannot be used in certain cardiac patients -High doses in elderly patients may cause confusion or urinary retention
Difenoxin	Motofen®	-Slows peristalsis	Narcotic, may be habit-forming if taken in doses larger than prescribed	-Similar to Lomotil, but is reported to be 2-4 times more effective
Tincture of Opium (historically known as Laudanum)		-Inhibits contraction of intestinal muscles, slowing down peristalsis and providing pain relief	Potent narcotic	-Dosing for tincture of opium should not be confused with dosing for Paregoric, which is much less potent

Anti-Spasmodics (Prescription)

Hyoscyamine	Levsin® Levbid® NuLev®	-Anti-spasmodic -Decreases cramping of stomach and intestines Anticholinergic (dries up secretions)	May cause drowsiness, urinary retention, and cardiac problems	-Taking antacids at the same time can decrease effectiveness -Can worsen GERD
Mebeverine	Colofac® Duspatal® Duspatalin®	-Antimuscarinic -Relaxes gut muscles at the cellular level -Normalizes small bowel motility		-Mainly used for treatment of IBS

Other (Prescription)				
Octreotide	Sandostatin®	Mimics somatostatin, which reduces the body's production of growth hormone, insulin, and glucagon	Can cause abdominal cramps and pain; can cause medically-induced diabetes; risk of bradycardia (slow heart rate)	-Used primarily for treatment of diarrhea and flushing with carcinoid syndrome
Bile Acid Sequestrants (Prescription)				
Colesevelam Cholestyramine Cholestipol	Welchol® Questran® Cholestid®	Binds bile acid, preventing reabsorption back into the gut; also used for lowering cholesterol	Risk of diarrhea, constipation, and gas. May bind fat-soluble Vitamins A, D, E, and K, requiring add'l supplementation	-May reduce bile-acid diarrhea -May interfere with medication absorption (e.g. digoxin)

Medications and Malabsorption

When food is malabsorbed, we anticipate medications and vitamin/mineral supplements will be malabsorbed as well. Patients spend hundreds or thousands of dollars on medications, only to have them pass through the entire digestive tract and into the stool without being absorbed into the body.

In my experience, the medications most frequently malabsorbed are pain medications, anti-depressants, and any extended-release or coated tablets. Patients will comment, "it seems like my anti-depressant isn't working anymore" or "my doctor keeps increasing my dosage, and the pain still isn't under control."

Please consult with your doctor or pharmacist. These are suggestions to maximize medication absorption:

- Switch medications to a chewable or liquid form. Be aware that many liquid medication preparations contain sorbitol
- Crush meds and mix with applesauce or yogurt
- Try a **transdermal patch** instead of pills, particularly for pain medications and hormone replacements

If your particular prescription medication does not come in one of these forms, you may benefit from using a **compounding pharmacy**. These specialized pharmacies modify medications for a patient's specific needs. Read more or locate a compounding pharmacy near you at: http://www.pccarx.com/patients/

Bulking Agents and Fibers

Bulking agents are fibers providing bulk and moisture to stools. Many people with IBS, either constipation-predominant (IBS-C) or alternating constipation/diarrhea (IBS-A), benefit from bulking agents to normalize stools. However, generally speaking, I do not recommend bulking agents for people with chronic diarrhea. In my experience, they tend to exacerbate symptoms of gas, bloating, and diarrhea. If you decide to try a bulking agent, I suggest Benefiber®, which tends to have fewer side effects. The following table lists some basic information about these fibers.

Common Fiber Supplements

Brand Name	Generic Name	Type of Fiber	Comments
Benefiber® (powder)		wheat dextrin (soluble)	
Metamucil® Konsyl Fiber®	psyllium husk	polysaccharide (contains both soluble and insoluble)	psyllium commonly causes gas and bloating in IBS
Citrucel®	methylcellulose	cellulose (claims to be 100% fermentable)	
FiberCon® (caplets) Equalactin®	calcium polycarbophil	calcium polycarbophil (claims to be 100% fermentable)	Best used by those suffering acute diarrhea or IBS. Works by equalizing the water balance of the intestines, absorbing 60 times its weight in water

The Bottom Line

Many over-the-counter and prescription medications list diarrhea as a common side effect. Your doctor or pharmacist can determine if another medication in the same category can be substituted without worsening your GI symptoms.

If you are taking a course of antibiotics, I recommend taking probiotics along with them to restore the population of good bacteria in your intestine.

In addition, there are many medications available to treat chronic diarrhea. Please discuss these options with your doctor or pharmacist.

If you have malabsorption, consider changing your medications to a liquid, patch, chewable, or crushed form to facilitate absorption.

Most of my patients with chronic diarrhea find that taking bulking agents such as Metamucil® actually worsens their GI symptoms. However, those with IBS alternating diarrhea/constipation may benefit from adding bulking agents to their daily regimen.

Chapter 10

Irritable Bowel Syndrome (IBS) and the FODMAP Diet

When I started having frequent diarrhea back in the 1980s (a long time ago!), my doctor put me through a battery of tests, including a barium enema, sigmoidoscopy, small bowel follow-through, and stool sample collection. Since all my tests were negative for inflammatory bowel disease, cancer, and infection, the doctor diagnosed me with **irritable bowel syndrome**, or **IBS**. In the past, IBS was often a **diagnosis of exclusion**, meaning if all medical tests came back negative, doctors would often label a patient with IBS, because they could not find anything specifically wrong.

In recent years, intense research has resulted in better ways to diagnose IBS. We now have diagnostic criteria which aid

IBS is common, affecting approximately 10-20% of the US population.

in making a diagnosis. IBS is currently defined as *the combination of abdominal pain and abnormal bowel habits (diarrhea, constipation or variable bowel movements) in the absence of other defined illnesses*.[26]

Studies in recent years have confirmed IBS is caused by many factors. Since each person is different, their particular cause of IBS may be different from another person. These are factors contributing to the development of IBS:

- *Intestinal dysmotility* The muscular movements in the intestines are either too fast or too slow.

- *Heightened brain-gut sensitivity* People with functional intestinal disorders, such as IBS, perceive pain differently. The brain does not properly regulate pain signals from the gut; those with IBS actually feel intestinal pain and pressure more intensely than people without IBS.

- *Psychosocial factors* Stressors affect movement and contractions of the GI tract, cause inflammation, or increase susceptibility to infection. (Chapter 7)

- *Impaired gut barrier* "Leaky gut syndrome." (Chapter 8)

- *Gut bacteria population* The effect of probiotics. (Chapter 8)

- *Food sensitivity* This will be discussed in Chapter 13.

- *Genetics* We are all born with genes that may predispose us to any of the above factors. Studies show that IBS tends to occur in families.

Irritable bowel syndrome is categorized into three sub-types:
- Constipation-predominant (IBS-C)
- Diarrhea-predominant (IBS-D)
- Alternating Constipation/Diarrhea (IBS-A), also known as pain-predominant

Treatment for IBS

There is no cure for IBS. However, there are many ways to manage the symptoms associated with this frustrating disorder. Many in the medical field have focused on treatment for IBS through medications. Meanwhile, the public has turned to self-help books and websites created by non-medical professionals, often promising miracle cures with extreme diets and a host of homeopathic supplements. I recommend steering clear of diets which promise a "cure" for IBS, although in my opinion, many of these books have valid suggestions which may improve your gastrointestinal symptoms.

Which treatments actually work for IBS? The answer is different for everyone, but in my experience, modifications in diet, stress management (Chapter 7), use of probiotics (Chapter 8), medications (Chapter 9), and exercise can have a huge impact.

Something New

As mentioned in Chapter 4, in recent years, Australian scientists studying functional gut disorders (such as IBS) discovered a relationship between fermentable carbohydrates like fructose and symptoms of gas, bloating, diarrhea, and even constipation. They coined a word for these particular carbohydrates: FODMAPs.

What Are FODMAPs?

The FODMAP acronym stands for:

Fermentable

Oligo-

Di-

Mono-saccharides

And

Polyols

Essentially, FODMAPs are carbohydrates and sugar alcohols which are poorly absorbed in the small intestine and rapidly fermented by gut bacteria. In simple terms, FODMAPs are certain dietary carbohydrates—sugars, starches, and fibers—which some people, especially those with IBS, cannot digest and absorb properly.

How Do FODMAPs Cause Diarrhea?

All FODMAPs cause IBS symptoms through the same mechanism:

- *Producing gas* as intestinal bacteria ferment the carbohydrate, causing abdominal pain and bloating
- *Pulling water* into the intestine by osmosis, causing osmotic diarrhea (Chapter 3)

Examples of FODMAPs

There are five main categories of FODMAPs; all are carbohydrates which are fermented quickly by the intestinal bacteria.

- *Galacto-oligosaccharides (GOS)* Complex carbohydrates found in beans, soy, and nuts

- *Fructose* Fruit sugar, high-fructose corn syrup, honey, and agave

- *Fructans* Complex carbohydrates found in wheat, onions, garlic, inulin, and fructo-oligosaccharides (FOS)

- *Lactose* Milk sugar

- *Polyols* Also called sugar alcohols, such as xylitol, mannitol, and sorbitol

Should I try the FODMAP diet?

Yes, it's definitely worth a try, especially if you have tried everything else. It is important to note that the FODMAP diet encompasses many of the principles mentioned in Chapter 4, plus several more. You may decide to try most or all of the strategies mentioned in this book prior to embarking on the FODMAP journey.

I highly recommend the book *IBS—Free at Last!* (second edition) written by Patsy Catsos, MS, RD. Her book outlines an elimination-type diet to determine which foods cause or aggravate the typical IBS symptoms of abdominal pain, gas, bloating, and diarrhea. Her approach is simple, straightforward, and research-based.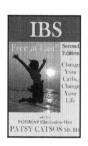

In addition, her website is a wealth of information on how to follow the FODMAP diet in "real" life. http://www.ibsfree.net/ibsfree_at_last/

Of all the strategies and treatments I have personally tried and professionally recommended for IBS, *the FODMAP diet has made the biggest improvements in my patients' symptoms.*

How Does the *IBS—Free at Last!* FODMAP Elimination Diet Work?

To start, all sources of FODMAPs are eliminated for two weeks. Good news—if the diet is going to work, you will feel better in the first two weeks! After the initial elimination phase, each category (galactans, fructose, fructans, lactose, polyols) is tested one by one to determine which types of FODMAPs produce symptoms, and how much can be eaten before symptoms begin.

The initial goal is to determine which FODMAPs cause your symptoms. Then, you need to monitor the quantities of FODMAPs consumed during a particular day. The overall goal is to maximize the number of foods you can eat as part of a healthy diet, while still preventing IBS symptoms.

Probiotics for IBS

Did you know there are probiotics developed and marketed especially for IBS? One example is VSL#3. You can read more on their website at: http://www.vsl3.com/

Some Prebiotics are FODMAPs

A word of caution: some prebiotics contain the fructans FOS and inulin, which are two of the FODMAP carbohydrates. You may just end up with more diarrhea!

The Bottom Line

IBS is a common cause of chronic diarrhea and other intestinal complaints. The FODMAP elimination diet is a relatively new concept that is worth trying for those with IBS. Research has demonstrated that some types of probiotics can improve IBS symptoms as well.

Chapter 11

Inflammatory Bowel Disease (IBD) and Ostomies

Inflammatory Bowel Disease (IBD)

IBD is a group of inflammatory conditions of the small and large intestine. The most common forms of IBD are Crohn's disease and ulcerative colitis (UC). Other types of colitis, such as lymphocytic, collagenous, and ischemic are also included.

Inflammatory bowel disease is an immune deficiency state, and is very different from irritable bowel syndrome, which was discussed in the last chapter. You can read more about Crohn's disease and UC, and how they are diagnosed and treated, on the Crohn's and Colitis Foundation website at: http://www.ccfa.org.

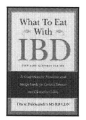

There are numerous diet books on the market for those with IBD; one I recommend is *What to Eat with IBD: A Comprehensive Nutrition and Recipe Guide for Crohn's Disease and Ulcerative Colitis* by Tracie Dalessandro, MS, RD, CDN.

Crohn's disease and ulcerative colitis are related diseases, but each has its own nutritional challenges. It is normal for a person with IBD to have periods of active disease called a **flare**, followed by quiescent times called **remission**.

Numerous websites and books promise an IBD cure with a special diet or supplement. Thus far, scientific studies have not supported these claims. However, as we will cover throughout this chapter, diet plays an important role in the treatment of both Crohn's disease and ulcerative colitis.

Crohn's Disease

Crohn's disease can affect the full length of the small bowel, but most commonly occurs in the last segment of the small intestine, the ileum. However, the disease can also be found in the colon, where it tends to occur in "patches". (In contrast, UC affects the entire colon.) The disease process causes deep ulcers in the intestinal lining, which can bleed. In severe cases, these ulcers can even perforate through the wall of the intestine, leading to a potentially dangerous abdominal infection.

When the small intestine is severely diseased, food may be eaten but does not get absorbed through the intestinal wall into the body. This can lead to malabsorption of important nutrients, vitamins, and minerals. It is common for those with moderate to severe active Crohn's disease to lose significant amounts of weight and suffer from chronic dehydration and malnutrition. If you have unintentionally lost more than seven percent of your body weight in three months, it is important to alert your doctor. Weight loss can be an indicator that you are not absorbing enough nutrients to maintain normal body functions.

Sometimes, those with Crohn's disease will need to take additional medications, such as steroids, during a flare. Other times, hospitalization with "gut rest" may be required, where no food or drink can be consumed by mouth. Instead, intravenous fluids may be administered to maintain hydration. In severe cases, if removing oral food and fluid does not help the patient's severe Crohn's symptoms, the doctor may prescribe total parenteral nutrition (TPN). This treatment bypasses the GI tract, delivering essential macronutrients, micronutrients, and other components through an intravenous line directly into the bloodstream. However, due to its high cost (over $1200 per day) and increased risk of infection, TPN is initiated only when the nutritional benefits outweigh the risks.

If the disease progresses and is unable to be controlled with medication and/or gut rest, surgery may be required. A patient who does not have adequate nutrition before surgery may have an extended recovery period and delayed healing.

Specific nutrients affected by active Crohn's disease are:

- Calcium (due to malabsorption in the upper small intestine) and iron (due to both malabsorption and blood loss from the bowel). Many of those with IBD have lactose intolerance and limit dairy intake.
- Magnesium and Vitamin B_{12} (due to ileal malabsorption).
- Sodium and potassium (due to excessive diarrheal losses).
- Protein, carbohydrate, and fat are commonly malabsorbed with severe Crohn's.

If your Crohn's disease is active, and you are concerned about your nutrition, please ask your doctor for a referral to a qualified registered dietitian. A dietitian who routinely works with IBD patients can provide a personalized meal plan and supplement suggestions. Below are recommendations I discuss with my Crohn's patients.

Nutrition Recommendations for a Crohn's Disease Flare

- *Increase calories and protein*, especially if you have had fevers or been on steroids as part of your medical management.

- If you continue to lose weight after increasing your food intake, you may need to *drink a specialized oral supplement*. These are similar to Ensure or Boost, but contain pre-digested carbohydrates, fats, and protein which get absorbed more easily across the intestinal wall into the body. I recommend Peptamen® with Prebio™. It comes in a mild vanilla flavor and can be used to supplement regular food intake.

- *Avoid high-fat foods*, which tend to increase malabsorption. If fat malabsorption remains a serious issue, a specialized fat supplement called medium chain triglyceride (MCT) oil may need to be substituted for regular long-chain fats in the diet. Peptamen® with Prebio™ also contains MCT oil.

- *Try the Easy-to-Digest Low-Fiber Diet* in Appendix C, especially if you have strictures (narrowing) and/or extensive Crohn's in the small intestine.

- *Avoid caffeine.*

- *Make sure you are adequately hydrated*, especially if you have over five bowel movements per day. (Chapter 17)

- If you are lactose intolerant, *add Lactaid tablets or switch to a Low-Lactose Diet* (Appendix D) until the flare has resolved.

- *Try the FODMAP elimination diet* (Chapter 10); it can be effective for those with IBD. However, this diet may not be appropriate for those with history of Crohn's strictures.

- If you been on antibiotics recently, *you may need probiotics.* (Chapter 8)

- Please *have your physician check a baseline bone scan, as well as your Vitamin D, folic acid, iron, Vitamin B_{12}, and magnesium levels for deficiencies,* especially if you have active disease in the ileum.

- *Recommended supplements:*

    - Daily adult multivitamin—chewable or liquid for better absorption

    - Calcium 1000-1200 mg per day

    - Vitamin D 2000 IU or more per day, or per MD

    - Folic Acid 800 mcg to 1 mg per day

    - Omega-3 fatty acids from fish oil capsules; get enteric-coated to prevent "fish burps." If **steatorrhea** occurs, discontinue the fish oil until disease is in remission

    - Additional supplements that may be recommended by your physician or dietitian are Vitamin B_{12}, iron, zinc, and magnesium

Nutrition Recommendations for Crohn's Disease in Remission

- The goal is to *regain weight and replace protein stores* that were depleted during the flare. Consume carbohydrates, proteins, and fats as tolerated.

- If you continue to lose weight even in remission, either you are not eating enough calories, or you are not truly in remission. Please discuss with your gastroenterologist.

- *Try eating some higher-fiber foods.* Focus on soluble fiber rather than insoluble fiber. (Chapter 4) Well-cooked and canned vegetables will be easier to tolerate at first. Add steamed and raw vegetables slowly back into the diet.

- *Begin a trial of lactose-containing foods.* Start with yogurt or white cheese, which are often easier to tolerate.

- If desired, *drink small amounts of caffeine as tolerated.*

- *Continue to take probiotics,* as directed on the bottle.

- *Recommended supplements*:
    - Daily adult multivitamin—chewable or liquid for better absorption
    - Calcium 1000-1200 mg per day
    - Vitamin D 2000 IU or more per day, or per MD
    - Folic Acid 800 mcg to 1 mg per day
    - Enteric-coated fish oil capsule (Omega-3's)
    - Additional supplements that may be recommended by your physician or dietitian are Vitamin B_{12}, iron, zinc, and magnesium

Ulcerative Colitis (UC)

Ulcerative colitis, unlike Crohn's disease, is found only in the colon. Since one of the main functions of the colon is water resorption, a diseased colon interferes with this process. Those with UC may suffer from watery or bloody diarrhea which varies from mild to severe. I have worked with UC patients who have 24 bowel movements a day!

Similar to Crohn's disease, severe blood loss from UC can lead to low iron levels, known as iron-deficiency anemia. Primary symptoms of anemia are weakness and tiredness, the same symptoms as dehydration. Your doctor can evaluate for anemia with a blood test. Those with anemia usually require iron supplementation. (Chapter 17) Occasionally, severe anemia will require a blood transfusion or intravenous iron infusion.

Nutrition Recommendations for Ulcerative Colitis Flare

- *Increase calories and protein,* especially if you have been on steroids as part of your medical management.
- *Try the Easy-to-Digest Low-Fiber Diet.* (Appendix C)
- *Make sure you are adequately hydrated,* especially if you have over five bowel movements per day. (Chapter 17)
- If you are lactose intolerant, *add Lactaid tablets or switch to the Low-Lactose Diet* (Appendix D) until the flare has resolved.
- *Try the FODMAP elimination diet* (Chapter 10); it can be effective for those with UC.
- If you been on antibiotics recently, *you may need probiotics.* (Chapter 8)

- *Recommended supplements*:
  - Daily adult multivitamin—chewable or liquid for better absorption
  - Calcium 1000-1200 mg per day
  - Vitamin D 2000 IU or more per day, as per your physician
  - Folic Acid 800 mcg to 1 mg per day
  - Enteric-coated fish oil capsule (Omega-3's)
  - Additional supplements that may be recommended by your physician or dietitian are iron and zinc

Nutrition Recommendations for Ulcerative Colitis in Remission

- The goal is to *regain weight and replace protein stores* that were depleted during flare. Consume carbohydrates, proteins, and fats as tolerated.
- *Try eating some higher-fiber foods*. Focus on soluble fiber rather than insoluble fiber. (Chapter 4) Well-cooked and canned vegetables will be easier to tolerate at first. Add steamed and raw vegetables slowly back into the diet.
- *Begin a trial of lactose-containing foods*. Start with yogurt or white cheese, which are often easier to tolerate.
- If desired, *drink small amounts of caffeine as tolerated*.
- *Continue to take probiotics*, as directed on the bottle.

- *Recommended supplements*:
  - Daily adult multivitamin—chewable or liquid preferred for better absorption)
  - Calcium 1000-1200 mg per day
  - Vitamin D 2000 IU or more per day, or per MD
  - Folic Acid 800 mcg to 1 mg per day
  - Enteric-coated fish oil capsule (Omega-3 's)
  - Additional supplements that may be recommended by your physician or dietitian are iron and zinc

Probiotics for IBD

I generally recommend one particular probiotic, VSL#3®, for my IBD patients. Unfortunately, scientific studies have favored the use of this probiotic for patients with UC or pouchitis over those with Crohn's disease. This probiotic contains a specialized formulation of eight strains of probiotic bacteria. Dosing varies from one to eight packets per day, determined by both the disease being treated and the number of stools per day. According to their website, maximum population of the gut takes place within 20 days.

More information can be found at http://www.vsl3.com/. Many patients with UC and IBS have less chronic diarrhea by using VSL #3. The major downside of using VSL #3 is the expense. However, some insurance carriers will cover the cost of this probiotic with a prescription.

J-pouch and Ileostomy

If you have had **j-pouch** or **ileostomy** surgery for IBD, these are my general nutrition recommendations:

Nutrition Recommendations for J-pouch or Ileostomy

- *Follow the Easy-to-Digest Low-Fiber Diet (Appendix C) for the first six weeks after surgery.*

- After that time, *begin reintroducing foods back into your diet,* such as whole grains, and fresh fruits and vegetables. Add one new food every two or three days. Use a journal to record your tolerance to each new food.

- *Reintroduce lettuce and vegetables with skins and seeds last.*

- From my experience with patients and advice from enterostomal therapy nurses, those with a j-pouch or ileostomy should *avoid mushrooms, corn, and popcorn.* They are not well-digested and increase risk for blockage of the stoma.

- Remember, just because you are *allowed* to eat a food, does not mean you *must* eat it. Many of my ostomy patients leave certain foods out of their diet, especially if they cause abdominal discomfort or gas.

- Due to high output from the stoma, *ileostomates need to consume greater amounts of fluids,* especially those containing both sodium and potassium (Chapter 17).

- *Any medications, vitamins, or minerals should chewable, crushed, liquid, or in a **transdermal patch*** to maximize absorption.

The Bottom Line

In addition to causing diarrhea, Inflammatory Bowel Disease can have a significant impact on your nutritional status and requires individualized care by a gastroenterologist and registered dietitian.

Chapter 12

Celiac Disease

Celiac Disease Defined

Celiac disease (CD) is an autoimmune disorder in which the body has a toxic reaction to **gluten**, the storage protein in the cereal grains *wheat*, *rye*, and *barley*. Current research indicates that CD is present in approximately 0.71 percent of the U.S. population[47]. Common symptoms of celiac disease include diarrhea, abdominal pain and gas, weight loss, unexplained infertility, neurologic conditions, unusual bleeding or anemia (due to vitamin/mineral deficiencies), and osteoporosis. There are numerous other symptoms which are not listed here.

How Do You Get Celiac Disease?

There are three factors in the development of celiac disease: genetic, environmental, and immunologic. First,

> Approximately 40% of the U.S. population is born with the genetic predisposition for CD.

a person must inherit specific genetic markers (DQ2 or DQ8) to get celiac disease. Next, the person with these genes experiences an environmental trigger or physical stressor. Some examples of environmental or physical stressors I have observed with my patients include:

- Emotional events—divorce, loss of a family member or close friend.
- Stress—at work, school, or home.
- Surgery or severe infection, especially if the infection required powerful antibiotics.

- Severe gastroenteritis (viral illness accompanied by vomiting and/or diarrhea) or "traveler's diarrhea" which never completely clears up.

Genetics + Environmental/Physical Stressor + Gluten in the Diet
=
Celiac Disease

Interestingly, not everyone who has the genetic markers develops celiac disease after a stressor event. One leading theory is that stressor events elicit a change in bacteria population in the gut, leading to **intestinal permeability** or **leaky gut syndrome.** (Chapter 8) When a protein such as gluten leaks from the inside the intestine into the tissue, it activates the immune response. Once the switch in the immune system is flipped "on," it changes how the body perceives gluten. So the next time the person ingests gluten, the body sees it as an invader.

After the disease has been triggered, the immune system attacks the finger-like absorptive lining (called **villi)** in the small intestine. Eating gluten causes the villi in the small intestine to flatten, and is called villous atrophy. Normal villi look like peaks and valleys, while the villi of someone with celiac disease looks more like low rolling hills.

Progression of Celiac Disease

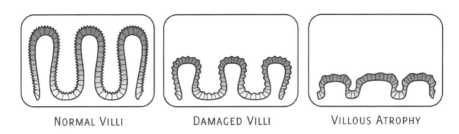

NORMAL VILLI   DAMAGED VILLI   VILLOUS ATROPHY

The villi constitute the main site of absorption in the small intestine. If they are damaged, *the body is unable to absorb key macro and micronutrients,* causing malnutrition.

Testing for Celiac Disease

A physician should diagnose celiac disease. He or she may begin with a screening blood test for CD, such as tissue transglutaminase antibodies (tTg IgA) and/or endomysial antibody (EMA). Both of these tests are highly sensitive and specific for celiac disease.

However, there can be false positive or negatives with blood tests. Therefore, experts in the celiac field recommend the "gold standard" method of diagnosis: an endoscopy with a small bowel biopsy.

What Is an Endoscopy with Biopsy?

After the patient is sedated, an endoscope, a small camera at the end of a flexible tube, is inserted through the mouth. As the endoscope is advanced through the esophagus, stomach, and duodenum, the gastroenterologist looks for abnormalities in the function and tissue of the digestive tract. Once the camera is in the duodenum, the doctor may biopsy, or remove, tissue samples with a small pincher, especially if the villi look abnormal.

Biopsy samples are sent to the lab and reviewed under the microscope by a pathologist. They are looking for flattened villi, as mentioned above, as well as specific inflammatory cells. Once a diagnosis of celiac disease is confirmed, the patient should meet with a registered dietitian to learn the principles of a strict, life-long, gluten-free (GF) diet.

Should I Try a Gluten-Free Diet Before Diagnosis?

Physicians and dietitians specializing in the treatment of CD recommend that people *do not* start the gluten-free diet until they have the small bowel biopsy. If you start this diet and choose to get tested later, you will likely have a false negative result. The small bowel will have healed up and blood tests may be in the normal range. In addition, villi will look at least somewhat healthy during endoscopy and on the pathology report.

Treatment for Celiac Disease

At the present time, *the only medical treatment for celiac disease is a life-long 100 percent gluten-free diet.* No wheat, rye, barley, kamut, spelt, triticale, malt, or contaminated grains. Only certified gluten-free grains are recommended; they are tested to be sure they contain less than 20 parts per million (ppm) of gluten. Certified GF grains are free from gluten contamination growing in the field, during transportation, storage, and finally, in processing.

What Is Gluten?

Gluten is the storage protein that gives bread its structure and elasticity, or stretchiness. If you have ever made your own bread, one of the steps is kneading the dough. If you pull it apart, you can see the gluten strings. Bread containing gluten also has a distinct texture when you chew it.

Why Follow the GF Diet for Celiac Disease?

If you took normal intestinal villi and spread them out flat, they would cover an area roughly the size of a tennis court. If you have untreated celiac disease (or are not following the GF diet closely), and the villi lose all their peaks and valleys, which can decrease the surface area to about the size of a table top! This means your body is unable to absorb all the nutrients it needs to maintain health.

Over time, malabsorption of nutrients leads to poor nutritional status and vitamin and mineral deficiencies. In addition, those with CD who still eat gluten have a higher risk of developing osteoporosis, other autoimmune diseases, and even some types of intestinal cancers. *The GF diet is one diet where there is no cheating allowed*. How much is considered cheating? Consuming enough wheat to cover your pinky fingernail each day is enough to result in ongoing intestinal damage.

Following a gluten-free diet can be challenging. Enlisting the help of a registered dietitian, your family, friends, and a local support group is essential. They can give you dos and don'ts on how to follow the GF diet at home, in restaurants, and when traveling. Gluten contamination can easily happen in restaurants with inappropriate food choices, and even in your own kitchen, sabotaging even the best of intentions.

Non-Celiac Gluten Sensitivity

For many years, when someone had a negative blood test and a negative small intestinal biopsy, that would confirm that this patient did not have celiac disease. They were advised to follow a regular diet, including gluten. End of story.

However, these same patients would often continue to have intestinal complaints for months or years. Some decided to follow a gluten-free diet on their own, and their symptoms disappeared. In recent years, scientists studied these patients and determined there is a diagnosis separate from celiac disease. They coined a new term: **non-celiac gluten sensitivity**. Since the knowledge base of gluten sensitivity is in its infancy, much is still unknown. For example, we do not yet know the long-term prognosis or progression, if there is one. The good news is that gluten sensitivity does not seem to affect the villi in the intestine, cause malabsorption, or increase risk of other autoimmune diseases. We anticipate new research in the future that will improve the diagnosis and treatment of this newly-identified disorder.

Diagnosing Non-Celiac Gluten Sensitivity

Testing for gluten sensitivity is a **diagnosis of exclusion**. The physician usually begins with the same blood tests used for celiac disease. Virtually all patients with celiac disease have the same genetic markers (DQ2 or DQ8). In patients with non-celiac gluten sensitivity, only about 50% have those same genetic markers. When AGA blood-testing is conducted, about 50% of patients with gluten sensitivity have a positive blood test for AGA-antibodies.

In patients with gluten sensitivity, intestinal biopsies are (virtually) normal. If celiac disease and IgE wheat allergy can be excluded, but the patient's symptoms are alleviated with a gluten-free diet, gluten sensitivity is suspected.

Treatment for Gluten Sensitivity

The treatment for non-celiac gluten sensitivity is a 100 percent gluten-free diet. An interesting observation by experts in the field is that minutes or hours after gluten exposure, *those with gluten sensitivity often report more intense symptoms (abdominal pain or diarrhea) than those with celiac disease.* In fact, these negative reactions sometimes make it easier for those with gluten sensitivity to fully adhere to the gluten-free diet.

Books and Research

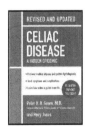 There are many excellent publications on the subject of celiac disease and the gluten-free diet. Some are well written and have accurate information, while others record more of a personal journey. One book I highly recommend is: *Celiac Disease: A Hidden Epidemic (Revised and Updated Edition 2010)* by Peter H. R. Green and Rory Jones. I jokingly call it the "Bible of Celiac Disease." Author Dr. Peter Green is a well-respected researcher and physician, who has published numerous studies and also founded The Celiac Disease Center at Columbia

132

University. He is dedicated to researching celiac disease, and is involved in direct patient care as well. Several other books I recommend:

Gluten-Free Diet: A Comprehensive Resource Guide—

Expanded and Revised

Edition

by Shelley Case, RD

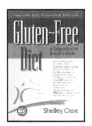

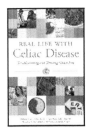

Real Life with Celiac Disease

by Melinda Dennis, MS, RD, LDN

and Daniel Leffler, MD, MS

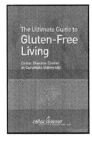

The Ultimate Guide to Gluten-Free Living

by Celiac Disease Center at Columbia University

Celiac Organizations

There are numerous organizations which support the celiac community in the United States. I highly recommend the Gluten Intolerance Group (GIG), based out of Seattle, Washington.

They have research-based information and resources for patients, their families, and the medical community. GIG has support groups all over the United States. www.gluten.net

Another support group is the Celiac Sprue Association. Their mission is "Celiacs Helping Celiacs." Find out more at www.csaceliacs.org

A list of other celiac websites and organizations can be found in Web Resources at the end of this book.

Gluten-Free Apps

Numerous smartphone apps have been created to help you make better gluten-free food choices.

- The Gluten Detective (from the Academy of Nutrition and Dietetics)
- Find Me Gluten Free
- Is that Gluten Free?
- Gluten Free
- Gluten Free Fast Food
- Gluten Free Recipes
- Gluten Freed—Gluten Free Dining
- Gluten Free Restaurant Card
- Gluten Free Restaurants

The Bottom Line

Undiagnosed celiac disease or non-celiac gluten sensitivity is a common cause of chronic diarrhea. Please see a physician for specific testing before embarking on a gluten-free diet. If diagnosed with one of these conditions, please consult with a registered dietitian, who can create a personalized nutrition plan with you. In addition, getting involved in local support groups significantly increases the success of following a life-long gluten-free diet.

Chapter 13

Food Allergies, Intolerances, and Sensitivities

Do you have any food allergies or intolerances? Do you know the difference? Medical professionals tend to like obvious diagnoses that fit into nice, neat boxes. Unfortunately, food allergies and intolerances are not always clear-cut, and can be challenging to diagnose and treat. We discussed lactose and fructose intolerance, two common causes of diarrhea, in Chapter 4. In this chapter, you will learn how diarrhea can also be a symptom of food allergy.

Food Allergy

When you hear the term **food allergy**, what is your first thought? Most people think of someone with a peanut allergy who has trouble breathing after an exposure. This is an example of the most severe, life-threatening allergic reaction, called **anaphylaxis**. However, there are many less-severe forms of food allergy.

Food allergy *involves a response from the body's immune system to a particular food protein.* The effects of food allergy occur in three main organ systems: the respiratory tract, skin, and digestive system. Symptoms may include hives, wheezing, itchy and watery eyes, sneezing, nasal discharge, nausea, vomiting, and diarrhea, which *typically occur within two hours of eating a particular food.* Headaches are a common allergic reaction to food as well, though they are not directly connected to the main allergenic organ systems.

Eight Most Common Food Allergens

Food allergies are more common in children than adults. Many children outgrow food allergies by age five.

The eight most common food allergens are listed below. These foods account for over 90 percent of all food allergies[51]:

- cow's milk and milk products

- eggs

- wheat

- soy

> According to the US Food and Drug Administration (FDA), over 160 foods can potentially cause allergic reactions[51].

- peanuts

- tree nuts (almonds, brazil nuts, cashews, hazelnuts, macadamia, pecans, pine nuts, pistachios, walnuts)

- fish

- shellfish (shrimp, prawns, lobster, crab, crayfish/ crawfish/crawdads) and mollusks (clams, mussel, oysters, scallops)

The food allergies that are the most likely to continue to adulthood are:

- peanuts

- tree nuts

- shellfish

- fish

> It is estimated that the prevalence of true food allergy in children under age five is up to 8%, and only 4% among adults[52].

The severity of allergic response differs from person to person and from allergen to allergen. In adults, shellfish exposure may cause anaphylaxis, while common symptoms of soy allergy include asthma and hives.

How Do Food Allergies Develop?

The mechanism causing food allergy is complicated, and is affected by genetics, diet, lifestyle and other environmental factors. People with a family history of food allergies, seasonal allergies, or asthma are at increased risk for developing food allergy.

This section will highlight key points to help you understand the basic physiology of how food allergies develop. If you wish to learn more about this complex topic, an excellent book for further reading is: *Dealing with Food Allergies. A Practical Guide to Detecting Culprit Foods and Eating a Healthy, Enjoyable Diet*, by Janice Vickerstaff Joneja, PhD, RD.

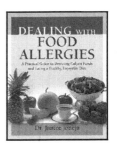

Every day, the immune system in the digestive tract must differentiate between healthy food and pathogenic bacteria, viruses, and chemicals. All foods contain molecules called **antigens**. Antigens that activate the immune system and have the potential to cause allergy are called **allergens,** which include pollen (from plants) and proteins (from food).

If an allergen is identified as an invader in your body, the immune system creates **antibodies** for that particular food. The next time you eat even small amounts that offending food, your body will recognize the food as a foreign substance, triggering an allergic reaction. Antibodies are also called **immunoglobulins (Ig)**, and consist of five subtypes, IgA, IgD, IgE, IgG, and IgM. **IgE** is the primary antibody when describing classic food allergy, especially anaphylaxis.

In an allergic response, symptoms may appear within minutes after coming in contact with a particular food, substance, or medication. This is because the body releases histamine, targeting a specific area of the body.

- An allergic response in the *lungs* is called asthma.
- An allergic response in *the nose* is called hay fever, or allergic rhinitis.
- An allergic response on the *skin* is called hives, or angioedema.
- An allergic response in the *gut* is called food allergy.
- A multi-system, life-threatening, *whole-body response* is called **anaphylaxis**.

Food Allergy Testing

To get properly diagnosed, it is best to visit an allergist/immunologist, a physician who specializes in identifying and treating allergies, asthma, and other immune system disorders.

Blood Tests

Typically, you will have an IgE blood test for food allergies. The results of the IgE blood test indicate the allergen levels for each food as low, moderate, high, or very high, based on a normal reference range. However, the laboratory tests are only valuable if the results correlate with symptoms for a particular food.

The doctor may recommend that you avoid any foods graded as moderate" or high reactivity on the IgE food allergy test. The downside to this approach is that the patient may avoid more foods than necessary. For non-anaphylactic reactions, an alternative method is to complete a single food challenge to determine if it is a true food allergy. Remove that particular food from the diet for several weeks, then re-introduce it and note any allergenic reactions. Food challenges for severe or anaphylactic food reactions (particularly in children) should be conducted under MD supervision in the medical office in case an allergic response requires immediate medical intervention.

Of note, foods with increased reactivity on an IgE blood test tend to cause symptoms in the respiratory tract or skin, rather than the digestive system.

Personal Story:

Our son, who has gastroesophageal reflux disease, had an IgE blood panel drawn to look for specific food allergies. The only food demonstrating moderate reactivity was hazelnuts. Although he eats hazelnuts infrequently, he does not have any noticeable reaction when he eats them. Therefore, he is not considered to be allergic to hazelnuts, and can continue to eat them. However, we will continue to monitor his tolerance to this food long-term.

Skin Tests

An allergist may also perform skin tests to confirm the presence of food allergies. As with other tests, there are false positives as well as false negatives. The allergist must combine the results of skin and blood tests with clinical symptoms to make an accurate diagnosis of food allergy.

Not all reactions are IgE mediated

To make it even more confusing, some reactions are non-IgE-mediated, such as celiac disease. This is in contrast to wheat allergy, which will demonstrate reactivity on an IgE blood test. Gluten activates the immune system by a different mechanism.

Diarrhea, as a symptom of food allergy, may present differently from other types of diarrhea discussed in this book. One difference is that the response is usually noted immediately after a meal. In addition, the watery diarrhea may contain blood, and be present with nausea, vomiting, hives, swelling of face, tongue, or throat, and/or wheezing at the same time.

Food Intolerance

In contrast to food allergy, **food intolerance,** also called non-allergic food hypersensitivity, is defined as *an adverse reaction to a food or food additive which does not involve the immune system.* Despite advances in medicine and science, the mechanisms of food intolerance are still poorly understood and are much harder to diagnose and manage than food allergy.

Carbohydrate Intolerance

The most common forms of food intolerance are to the carbohydrates lactose and fructose. (Chapter 4) Symptoms are generally confined to the digestive system, causing nausea, vomiting, gas, bloating, belching, diarrhea, or constipation. However, migraine headaches can also be an indicator of food intolerance.

Other Intolerances Associated with Diarrhea

Another possibility is intolerance to lesser-known groups of compounds called biogenic amines. The symptoms associated with gastrointestinal (and usually skin and respiratory) distress from biogenic amines include:

- *Histamine*: Found in fermented foods such as sauerkraut and soy products, cheese, alcoholic beverages, and vinegars; also occurs naturally in strawberries, egg whites, and shellfish

- *Benzoates*: Found in baked goods, pickles, margarine, chewing gum, fruit preserves, and as a flavoring agent in some beverages; also occurs naturally in berries such as raspberries and strawberries, some spices, prunes, and tea

Food Intolerance Testing

Currently there are only a few tests available for food intolerances. **Hydrogen breath tests** (Chapter 4) used to diagnose lactose and fructose intolerance are expensive and not widely available, so their use is limited. Many people find that an elimination diet or food challenge is the most effective way to determine if they are intolerant to a particular food.

Case Study:

Several years ago, I had a patient with chronic diarrhea (six or more times a day) who tried many different diets, including a strict elimination diet. Through the process, he discovered he did not have lactose intolerance or gluten sensitivity. Instead, he was allergic to corn, including whole corn, corn syrup, and high-fructose corn syrup, which is found in many processed foods. Once he began avoiding all corn, his diarrhea disappeared.

Food Sensitivity

If a person has nausea, vomiting, abdominal pain, or diarrhea after eating a particular food, it may be unclear whether the reaction is due to a food allergy or intolerance. Even though the body's mechanisms for these two conditions are very different, as you have seen, some of the symptoms overlap. Without a clear diagnosis, the reaction may be referred to as **food sensitivity**.

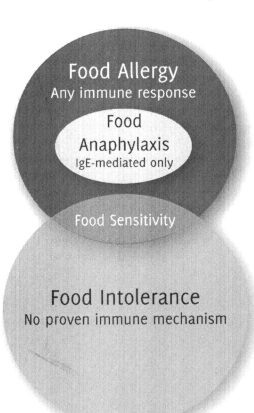

Symptoms of Food Intolerance vs. Food Allergy

Symptoms	Food Intolerance	Food Allergy
Sneezing/nasal discharge		☑
Itchy, watery eyes		☑
Asthma/shortness of breath		☑
Tongue swelling		☑
Anaphylaxis/throat tightening		☑
Hives/itching/swelling/rash		☑
Oral allergy syndrome		☑
Headaches	☑	☑
Indigestion/nausea/vomiting	☑	☑
Gas/bloating/abdominal pain/belching	☑	☑
Diarrhea	☑	☑
Constipation	☑	

Food Allergy Treatment

Once a food allergy has been identified, the only treatment is to completely avoid eating or coming in contact with the offending food, since symptoms can worsen over time. Unfortunately, taking probiotics or allergy shots will *not* prevent or treat an allergic reaction to a food.

Furthermore, if you have been diagnosed with a food allergy and have experienced severe whole-body reactions, it is advisable to carry injectable epinephrine (called an EpiPen®) with you at all times. You should be educated on how and when to use it in case of an accidental exposure.

Food Intolerance Treatment

Foods causing lactose or fructose intolerance do not need to be avoided entirely, since the immune system is not involved. Rather, intake is managed depending on your personal tolerance. For example, if you have lactose intolerance, you may be able to drink small amounts of milk. Studies have shown you may be able to increase your tolerance to lactose over time, by slowly increasing your daily intake. Fructose intake must be monitored in combination with other FODMAPs.

In contrast, food or additives causing other adverse reactions should be removed from the diet entirely. The goal is to control symptoms long-term.

Food Is Not the Culprit

When discussing food allergy and intolerance, there is one important point to remember: *food does not in itself cause allergy or intolerance*. Rather, it is our body's *inappropriate reaction* toward a particular food or substance.

The Bottom Line

Food sensitivities can be a potential cause of diarrhea and should be evaluated. It is important to understand that the purpose of this book is not to diagnose food allergy or intolerance; these must be diagnosed by a physician or allergist. The ultimate goal in treating food sensitivities is to maximize what you *can* eat, rather than eliminating entire food groups out of fear of having a reaction.

Chapter 14

Pancreatic Insufficiency

Pancreatic Insufficiency

In Chapter 2 we discussed normal intestinal anatomy and physiology. Sometimes, the pancreas does not produce enough enzymes to break down the fats, carbohydrates, and/or proteins from food. This condition is called **pancreatic insufficiency**, and can occur after previous surgeries, diseases, procedures, or radiation treatment.

Essentially, the food passes through the entire digestive system and out of the body without being broken down for absorption. Diarrhea is a frequent symptom of pancreatic insufficiency, as well as steatorrhea, weight loss, edema, anemia, fatigue, gas, and abdominal distention.

Causes of Pancreatic Insufficiency

- Cancers and tumors, such as biliary or pancreatic
- Celiac disease
- Crohn's disease
- Chronic pancreatitis
- Cystic fibrosis
- Radiation enteritis
- Surgery, such as a Whipple procedure, or gastric bypass
- Whipple's disease (a rare infectious disease caused by a bacterium, Tropheryma whipplei, which causes malabsorption)
- Zollinger-Ellison syndrome

Why Is Diagnosis of Pancreatic Insufficiency Important?

Left untreated, pancreatic insufficiency can eventually lead to malnutrition and nutrient deficiencies, particularly fat-soluble vitamins A, D, E, and K.

How Do I know if I Have Pancreatic Insufficiency?

A physician who suspects pancreatic insufficiency may order a fecal fat test to rule out fat malabsorption. For this test, you must consume over 100 grams of fat each day, for three days straight. (Keep in mind a stick of butter is 92 grams!) You must also collect all your bowel movements in a container, and then submit them for analysis. Results:

- If you have two to seven grams of fat in your stool per 24 hours, you *do not* have fat malabsorption.
- More than seven grams of fat in your stool per 24 hours means you *do* have fat malabsorption.

Years ago, gastroenterologists conducted this test more frequently; now, it is less commonly ordered. Today, many physicians will write a prescription for replacement pancreatic enzymes based on medical history alone.

What Is the Treatment for Pancreatic Insufficiency?

Once diagnosed, typical treatment involves taking oral **pancreatic enzymes** with food to replace the enzymes (protease, amylase, lipase) the pancreas is not producing.

How Are Pancreatic Enzymes Replaced?

Pancreatic enzymes are available with a doctor's prescription. Examples of prescription pancreatic enzymes are Creon® and Pancreaze®.

Some naturopathic doctors offer similar enzymes without a prescription. However, these are not recommended. Over-the-counter (OTC) pancreatic enzymes are not regulated in the same way as prescription medications. The amount of viable (living) enzymes in OTCs can vary greatly from batch to batch, making it extremely difficult to know how many to take at each meal. Another consideration—medical insurance *will* cover pancreatic enzymes by prescription, while it *will not* cover OTC or naturopath-prescribed enzymes.

What Do Pancreatic Enzymes Look Like, and How Do I Take Them?

Pancreatic enzymes are oral capsules containing enzymes, not a medication. They are similar to the lactase enzymes taken for lactose intolerance. Pancreatic enzymes are taken *with* food or snacks to break down fats, proteins, and carbohydrates so they can be absorbed into the body. You must change the dose based on how much fat or protein there is in the meal. Generally, two or three enzyme capsules are taken at meals, and one or two with snacks. Some meals require more enzymes, some snacks need fewer.

Years ago, I heard a physician speak on this topic, and she recommended one pancreatic enzyme per each five to seven grams of fat in a meal. I still use this guideline as a starting point for my patients. From there, we work up or down on the dose depending on their symptoms.

Are There any Foods or Drinks I Can Have without Taking Pancreatic Enzymes?

In general, pancreatic enzymes are *not* needed for coffee, tea, fruit juice, oral rehydration solutions (Chapter 17), popsicles, soda, or fruit (if eaten alone, without other foods containing protein or fat.)

The Bottom Line

Pancreatic insufficiency is not a frequent cause of diarrhea, but it should be considered if you have any of the diagnoses listed above. Treating this condition with simple pancreatic enzymes can result in improved absorption of nutrients, and consequently, less diarrhea.

Chapter 15

Esophageal, Stomach, and Intestinal Surgery

What happens to your ability to digest nutrients after surgery on your GI tract? It depends on which portion of your anatomy was altered. This chapter will move through the digestive tract, discussing different surgical procedures and how each affects digestion and absorption.

Surgical History

I will begin by making one important recommendation: if you have had abdominal surgery, please get a copy of both your surgery and pathology reports. It may be extremely helpful for a dietitian or doctor several years down the road to have a written copy of the exact procedure for reference. Information should include:

- What part(s) were removed (**resected**)?
- Length of the section removed.
- What was left unaffected?
- Was the digestive system re-routed? Can your physician draw of picture of what your new anatomy looks like?
- Any complications?
- Results of the pathology report.
- Any follow up surgeries?

Esophagus

As reviewed in Chapter 2, the function of the esophagus is to deliver food from the mouth to the stomach. With esophageal cancer, the surgeon will generally remove the diseased portion of the esophagus along with the esophageal sphincter in a procedure called an **esophagogastrectomy**. The remaining esophagus is re-attached to the stomach. Diarrhea is not usually a side effect of this surgery. Occasionally, the diseased esophagus may be replaced with a small section of your own colon or small intestine, called a neo-esophagus. In this case, the patient may have post-surgical diarrhea similar to a typical bowel resection.

Stomach

Stomach cancer or severe stomach ulcers may require the removal of part (**subtotal gastrectomy**) or all (**total gastrectomy**) of the stomach. Gastric bypass surgery for morbid obesity (Roux-en-Y) is another example of stomach surgery. Resection of the lower portion of the stomach usually includes the **pyloric valve**, which regulates the speed of food leaving the stomach.

Whipple Procedure

A **Whipple procedure**, also known as a pancreaticoduodenectomy, is a surgical procedure used to remove cancerous tumors of the pancreas, common bile duct, or duodenum near the pancreas. The most common technique consists of the removal of the lower portion of the stomach, the first and second part of the duodenum, the head of the pancreas, the common bile duct, and the gallbladder.

In more recent years, a modified version of this surgery involves leaving the stomach and pyloric valve intact (pylorus-sparing Whipple procedure). These patients have far fewer issues with chronic diarrhea.

Since part of the pancreas is removed during surgery, patients undergoing either type of Whipple procedure may need to take pancreatic enzymes with their food. (Chapter 14)

Other Nutritional Concerns after Whipple Procedure or Gastric Bypass

Unintentional weight loss often occurs after stomach surgery due to numerous issues, including poor appetite, inadequate caloric intake, malabsorption (from inadequate pancreatic enzymes and/or increased motility), and chronic diarrhea.

If you have had a Whipple procedure or gastric bypass, you may have difficulty absorbing calcium and/or iron because both are absorbed in the duodenum. Long-term malabsorption of calcium can result in softening of the bones, called **osteopenia**. Inadequate absorption of iron from the duodenum can lead to iron-deficiency anemia. After either of these surgeries, you will also need ongoing Vitamin B_{12} supplementation with periodic blood work to monitor your B_{12} status. Calcium, iron, and Vitamin B_{12} supplementation will be covered in Chapter 17.

Dumping Syndrome

Regardless of which specific surgery was performed, loss of the pyloric valve commonly results in a phenomenon called **dumping syndrome**.

Symptoms occur when sugary food and liquids are released from the small stomach pouch into the small intestine too quickly. This overloads the capacity of the small intestine to handle sugar. Cutting back or avoiding sweet foods is effective in reducing dumping syndrome diarrhea. Dumping syndrome has an early and a late phase.

In the early phase, dumping syndrome occurs about 30 to 60 minutes after eating. Symptoms include:

- flushed feeling
- rapid heart rate
- nausea or vomiting
- abdominal cramping
- urgent (osmotic) diarrhea

Late phase dumping syndrome occurs one to three hours after eating. Symptoms are caused by a surge of insulin, which drops blood sugar quickly (hypoglycemia):

- flushed feeling
- rapid heart rate
- dizziness, fainting
- mental confusion

Eating Strategies after Stomach Surgery

If you have had stomach surgery (with removal of the pyloric valve), dumping syndrome can be minimized by altering how you eat and drink. This modified way of eating slows down food movement through the digestive system, allowing more time for absorption of nutrients.

Here are the recommendations for eating after stomach surgery:

- *Six small feedings per day.* Due to the stomach's smaller capacity, you will feel fuller faster. Remember to chew your food well. This puts less strain on the stomach to grind your food.

- *Sugary, sweet, or rich foods should be avoided, since these aggravate dumping syndrome.* Some people are very sensitive to sugar after stomach surgery and cannot tolerate it in any amount. These are typically the hyperosmolar foods and drinks mentioned in Chapter 4 and are listed in the following table.

Examples of Sugary Foods That Increase Dumping Syndrome	
white sugar	desserts (cakes, cookies, pies)
brown sugar	pastries
honey	ice cream
agave	jam
pancake syrup	concentrated (very sweet) juices
flavoring syrup	regular soda
corn syrup	candy and gum
**Alternative sweeteners such as stevia, Splenda®, NutraSweet®, Sweet'N Low®, or Sugar Twin® are acceptable substitutes. They do not aggravate dumping.	

- *Stop drinking liquids 15 minutes before a meal; do not resume drinking until about 30-60 minutes after eating.* This slows down the passage of food through the digestive tract, allowing better nutrient absorption and decreasing the risk of dumping syndrome. Since it is important to stay well hydrated, sip water or unsweetened, non-carbonated, decaffeinate liquids throughout the day. (Chapter 17)

- *Start with a low-fiber diet and add fiber back gradually.* Choose foods from the Easy-to-Digest Low-Fiber Diet in Appendix C. Gradually add one new food from the "avoid list" every three or four days and enter it in your journal. If you tolerate that food, try a new one. Gradually add new foods as tolerated.

- *Avoid caffeine.* Caffeine, found in regular coffee, tea, colas, chocolate, and energy drinks, speeds up intestinal motility and can exacerbate diarrhea.

- *Avoid carbonation.* Carbonation can increase intestinal gas and discomfort.

- *Evaluate yourself for lactose intolerance.* Lactose intolerance (Chapter 4) is common after surgeries involving the stomach and first portion of the small intestine, called the duodenum.

- *Be patient.* Your body will slowly adapt to its "new" way of digestion. There may be foods that you do not tolerate in the beginning, but you may tolerate them weeks or months later. If you have an intolerance of a certain food, write it in your food journal. Try it again later to see if there is an improvement.

Vitamins, Minerals, Medications, and Supplements after Stomach Surgery

- Your diet after surgery is often inadequate in vitamins and minerals due to the smaller quantities of food you are consuming. I recommend *taking a liquid or chewable vitamin/mineral supplement daily.*

- You may also need *1000-1200 mg of calcium per day*, split into two different doses for better absorption. Try chewable Tums®, Viactive® Calcium Chews, or liquid calcium. Ask your physician if you need additional iron. (Chapter 17)

- If more than one third of the lower portion of your stomach is removed, you will need to *supplement Vitamin B_{12} for the rest of your life.* You can take Vitamin B_{12} with a daily under-the-tongue supplement (available over-the-counter), weekly nasal spray, or a monthly shot. Please consult your physician for the proper dose. (Chapter 17)

- If you are unable to obtain enough calories from food, *you may need an oral nutritional supplement.* I recommend Optisource®, or Carnation® Instant Breakfast Essentials™ No Sugar Added (if you tolerate lactose), which are less likely to cause dumping syndrome. *Note:* Oral supplements, such as Ensure®, Boost®, and Resource Breeze®, are high in osmolality, which can aggravate dumping. Another option is to dilute the supplement and sip small amounts, gradually increasing the volume to see if you can tolerate it.

Small Intestine

There are a number of conditions requiring **resection,** or removal, of the small intestine, including:

- Ulcers

- Carcinoid syndrome

- Crohn's disease

- Malignant and benign tumors

- Small bowel obstruction

- Ischemia (loss of blood flow, which can cause a section of bowel to "die")

- Meckel's diverticulum

Effect of Resection on Digestion

In Chapter 2 you learned there are three separate segments of the small intestine: the duodenum, the jejunum, and the ileum. The intestinal tract has an amazing ability to adapt; if the duodenum or the jejunum are removed, the ileum can take over their absorptive functions. However, the duodenum and jejunum are much less efficient at assuming the functions of the ileum. If the ileum is removed, the patient will likely have more side effects, including chronic diarrhea.

It is important to know whether or not your **ileocecal valve** was removed during surgery. This one-way valve's function is to keep bacteria from refluxing back into the small bowel. If this happens, it can lead to **small intestinal bacterial overgrowth** (SIBO), a condition that typically requires periodic antibiotic treatment. We will discuss SIBO in more detail in the next chapter.

The All-Important Ileum

The last segment of the small intestine, the ileum, has several important functions, including reabsorbing bile salts. (Chapter 2) Bile salts are important for the efficient absorption of fats and fat-soluble vitamins. A portion of the body's bile salts are reabsorbed from the ileum several times each day and then recycled back into the body to be used again. So, if a large portion of the ileum is removed, bile salts will not get properly recycled. The total body pool of bile salts eventually gets too low, worsening fat malabsorption. Without the ileum, extra bile salts arriving in the colon cause bile salt diarrhea. (Chapter 16)

In addition, the ileum is the site of magnesium and Vitamin B_{12} absorption. If most or all of the ileum is resected:

- Bile salt diarrhea may require a medication called a bile acid sequestrant, called cholestyramine. (Chapter 9)
- Low magnesium absorption may require supplementation. This is challenging, because taking oral magnesium can actually cause more diarrhea! Some people require periodic IV magnesium infusions. (Chapter 17)
- Vitamin B_{12} may need replacement, since the Vitamin B_{12}/intrinsic factor complex will be affected. (Chapter 17)

Short Bowel Syndrome

If too much of either the small or large intestine is removed, damaged, or dysfunctional, there may not be enough remaining bowel to absorb all the nutrients required by the body. This complex condition is called **short bowel syndrome (SBS)**.

SBS requires intensive nutritional monitoring by a medical team, including physicians, dietitians and pharmacists familiar with the potential complications and treatments.

Long-term complications of short bowel include:

- Inadequate carbohydrate and protein absorption
- Fat malabsorption
- Vitamin/mineral deficiencies
- Weight loss
- Chronic dehydration
- Osteoporosis, anemia
- Small bowel overgrowth
- Chronic diarrhea

More information and support for patients with SBS can be found at:

http://www.shortbowelfoundation.org/

http://shortbowelsupport.com/default.htm

http://www.oley.org/index.html

If an adult or child with short bowel syndrome cannot absorb enough nourishment to maintain normal body functions, the doctor or dietitian may order **total parenteral nutrition (TPN).** With TPN, nutrients are broken down into glucose (carbohydrates), amino acids (proteins), and lipids (fats) and combined with other vitamins, minerals, and medications. These ingredients are mixed in a sterile laboratory and placed in a bag. The bag of TPN is delivered to the patient, then pumped into the body through a special intravenous line called a PICC line. TPN can provide all the nutrition a patient needs, without having to eat. However, some patients choose to eat "recreationally," accepting side effects of dehydration and chronic diarrhea.

If the digestive system can still absorb some nutrition, the doctor or dietitian may order **tube feeding (TF).** In TF, a specialized pre-made formula is pumped through a small tube directly into the stomach or small bowel, providing all necessary nutrition. The tube may go through the nose and stomach to and deliver nutrition into the small intestine. Or a tube may be surgically placed in the stomach or small intestine. The formulas used for SBS patients resemble a can of Ensure®, except they are made specifically for tube feeding. Those with SBS may need TF formulas created for especially for malabsorption; these contain pre-digested carbohydrates, proteins, and fats that are easier to digest than regular food. Tube feeding can provide all the nutrition a patient needs, or can supplement the food they are already eating.

Another option to TPN or tube feeding is to *drink* the specialized malabsorption tube feeding formulas, although they are not particularly tasty. An example of one of these formulas is vanilla-flavored Peptamen® with Prebio™ made by Nestlé Nutrition. This option can be discussed with your doctor or dietitian.

Colon
Total Colectomy with Ileorectal Anastomosis
Chapter 2 described the main functions of the colon: completing carbohydrate digestion, and water and electrolyte re-absorption.

Sometimes, all or part of the entire large intestine must be surgically removed, a procedure called a **colectomy**. Reasons for a colectomy include:

- Inflammatory bowel disease, such as ulcerative colitis or Crohn's disease
- Familial adenomatous Polyposis (FAP)
- Diverticulosis or diverticulitis
- Colon or rectal cancer
- Bowel infarction (when bloodflow to the bowel is lost, and the bowel "dies")
- Toxic megacolon (usually resulting from clostridium difficile)
- Trauma
- Blockage, either internal from a tumor, or external from scar tissue from previous surgeries
- Bleeding

When the large intestine is removed, your ability to finish digesting carbohydrates and re-absorb fluid is compromised. The Easy-to-Digest Low-Fiber Diet (Appendix C) is effective in decreasing diarrhea after a colectomy. For others, the FODMAP diet approach (Chapter 10) can target which specific fermentable carbohydrates are aggravating GI symptoms. While a few of my patients have found adding bulk-forming fibers such as Metamucil® or Benefiber® decreases diarrhea, many complain that it simply worsens their intestinal symptoms. If you have a j-pouch or ileostomy, nutritional recommendations were provided in Chapter 11.

It takes approximately six to twelve months for the body to fully heal and adapt after intestinal surgery. Without the entire colon for water resorption, diarrhea is common. Some of my patients benefit from using medication such as loperamide (Imodium®) or diphenoxylate (Lomotil®) to slow down the motility of the intestinal tract, allowing more time for fluids to get absorbed back into the body.

The following are nutritional questions to consider for patients who have ongoing diarrhea after a colectomy:

- Exactly what surgery was performed? Is the ileocecal valve intact? Is your ongoing diarrhea related to SIBO? (Chapter 16)

- Are you losing so much fluid that you are chronically dehydrated? Replacing fluids containing sodium and potassium is extremely important. (Chapter 17)

- Have you discussed with your doctor the need to add medications specifically for diarrhea? (Chapter 9)

- Are your medications malabsorbed? Do you need to change them to a different form to ensure absorption? (Chapter 9)

Bowel Obstructions

After one or more abdominal surgeries, some people form scar tissue (adhesions) inside the abdominal cavity. Over time, this scar tissue can wrap itself around the intestine, causing a partial or complete **bowel obstruction**. Tumors inside and outside the intestinal wall, as well as strictures from Crohn's disease, can also cause bowel obstructions. Some bowel obstructions resolve on their own (the bowel becomes "unkinked"), while others require surgery. Many times, doctors do not want to perform another operation to release the adhesions, because more scar tissue may be formed in the process.

If you were to look at the inside of the intestinal tract during a partial blockage, you would see a very narrow opening, barely large enough for food to get by. (I have had patients with an opening only the size of a pencil eraser!) Many of these patients actually have chronic diarrhea, because only liquids can pass by the blockage. Food can get stuck, worsening the obstruction.

I had patients with chronic bowel obstructions who were readmitted to the hospital several times after food got stuck. I put them on the Easy to Digest Low-Fiber Diet in Appendix C. Once all potential blockage foods were removed from the diet, they had fewer bowel obstructions, and therefore fewer hospitalizations.

The Bottom Line

The digestive system, from the mouth to the anus, is intended to work as a single continuous unit. Therefore, any type of surgery will alter how your body breaks down and absorbs nutrients. Targeting the specific affected areas is important in managing the type of diarrhea you have and determining how to make changes to the nutrition going into your body. Partnering with a knowledgeable medical team, including a registered dietitian, is the key to long-term nutritional management.

Chapter 16

Other Causes of Diarrhea—Hormones, Serotonin, Bile-Acids, Cancer Treatment, Small Intestinal Bacterial Overgrowth, Running, and Gas

Female Hormones and Diarrhea

If you are a woman, you may find your diarrhea coincides with your menstrual cycle, due to the increased levels of the hormones progesterone and estrogen. As these hormones peak, usually during the first two days of menses, the colon muscles relax, causing diarrhea.

Hormone fluctuations can also lead to loose stools during menopause. In addition, if women take herbs with phytoestrogens (such as flaxseeds) to control hot flashes, common side effects include-—what else?—gas, bloating, and diarrhea.

Interestingly, in balloon distension studies (where a balloon is inserted into the rectum and inflated), women with IBS are more sensitive to gut pain during their menses[27]. While considered completely normal, monthly diarrhea can be very frustrating. You may find some simple dietary changes, such as decreasing insoluble fiber intake or caffeine for a few days each month, may be of great benefit.

Some patients report they have more diarrhea (or constipation) when they are taking birth control pills or have an IUD implanted. Hormones affect us all differently.

Vasoactive Intestinal Peptide (VIP) and Diarrhea

Vasoactive intestinal peptide (VIP) is a hormone normally found in the brain, gut, and pancreas. One of its functions is to relax smooth muscle in the intestine. Excess secretion of VIP is known to cause secretory diarrhea. Vasoactive intestinal peptide tumors or VIPomas typically begin in the pancreas and secrete high levels of VIP. Symptoms include crampy, watery, high output diarrhea which can quickly lead to dehydration and dangerously low sodium and potassium levels. VIPomas are rare and are diagnosed with blood tests and CT scans. Long-term treatment involves removing the tumor and taking medications such as octreotide. (Chapter 9)

To my knowledge, patients with these conditions do not need to follow a specific diet. However, if part of the pancreas has been surgically removed, the diet principles for pancreatic insufficiency may be appropriate. (Chapter 14)

Serotonin and Diarrhea

When you hear the word **serotonin**, you probably connect it with sleep. Serotonin is a chemical neurotransmitter involved in the regulation of:

- sleep
- temperature
- pain
- mood enhancement
- appetite suppression

> IBS may be affected by changes in serotonin levels.

In fact, roughly 90 percent of your body's serotonin is found in the **enterochromaffin cells** of the gastrointestinal tract. Why is this important? If your food contains a toxin or irritant, the enterochromaffin cells release serotonin, stimulating the gut to move the food through faster and causing diarrhea. So, if you are taking prescription or over-the-counter medications to enhance serotonin, assist with sleep, or suppress appetite, you may actually be causing *more diarrhea*. In the GI tract:

- High serotonin levels = diarrhea
- Low serotonin levels = constipation

Those with IBS-diarrhea predominant (IBS-D) may be prescribed Lotronex®. This medication blocks the sites of action for serotonin in the body, effectively decreasing serotonin levels and lessening diarrhea.

Carcinoid Syndrome

Carcinoid syndrome is a group of symptoms caused by slow-growing tumors of the **enterochromaffin**

> About 70% of carcinoid tumors are found in the GI tract[67].

cells in the small intestine, colon, appendix, and lungs. These cells secrete large quantities of serotonin, which causes flushing (of the face, hands, or upper chest), shortness of breath, transient abdominal pain, and diarrhea. In carcinoid syndrome, *nocturnal or nighttime diarrhea is a common symptom*. In contrast, in those with IBS, diarrhea episodes usually occur during the day.

Initial medical treatment for carcinoid syndrome involves removing or shrinking the tumor cells. Sometimes, the tumors cannot be completely removed, so carcinoid symptoms are managed long-term through medications and diet changes.

Diet for Carcinoid Syndrome

Basic diet recommendations for carcinoid syndrome include avoiding aged cheese, wine, alcohol, avocado, some nuts, and spicy foods. There are additional nutritional considerations for carcinoid syndrome that are outside the scope of this book. It is important for anyone with this condition to work with a supportive medical team, including a doctor, pharmacist, and registered dietitian.

Chronic Idiopathic Bile Acid Diarrhea

Chronic idiopathic bile acid diarrhea is also called **bile acid** or **bile salt malabsorption**. Recent research indicates the condition is not caused by malabsorption; rather, it is a result of *excess production of bile* by the liver.

In normal physiology, bile is produced by the liver and then stored in the gallbladder. Bile acids are one component of bile. In typical digestion, bile is released from the gallbladder through the common bile duct, to meet up with the food in the small intestine, where the bile assists with fat digestion.

Once the bile acids reach the ileum, about 90 percent is reabsorbed back into the body to be used again. This recycling process is completed about six to eight times per day. If you have excess bile acid secretion, the body is unable to recycle all the acid back into the system. When these surplus bile acids reach the colon, excess water is pulled into the bowel, causing osmotic diarrhea. Some people with this condition may have up to 10 watery diarrhea episodes per day.

Treatment for bile acid diarrhea consists of binding the excess bile salts so they can be excreted in the stool. Cholestyramine, colestipol and colesevelam are all generic brands of bile salt-binding medications proven to be effective in treating this condition.

At this time, there are no specific diet recommendations for bile acid diarrhea. However, in combination with medications, moderating fat intake may be a place to start.

Habba Syndrome

Habba syndrome is a condition where *the gallbladder releases bile incorrectly*, causing bile acid diarrhea. Habba syndrome may be diagnosed by a gastroenterologist with a specialized gallbladder scan. Similar to bile acid diarrhea, treatment involves using bile acid-binding medications to bind the excess bile, which is then excreted in the stool. No specific changes in diet have been proposed.

Cancer Treatment and Diarrhea

It is common to have diarrhea during chemotherapy treatment. Certain types of medications and chemo drugs are known to have diarrhea as a primary complication or side effect. While the diet principles presented in earlier chapters can be beneficial, short-term diarrhea due to chemotherapy must sometimes take its course.

Some people find they have temporary sensitivities to foods. (Chapter 4) If this is you, remove these foods, at least until the chemotherapy treatment is complete or your symptoms have abated. A long discussion for the treatment of diarrhea related to cancer treatment is outside the scope of this book. I highly recommend you consult with a registered dietitian who specializes in oncology (cancer) nutrition.

Small Intestinal Bacterial Overgrowth (SIBO)

Another cause of chronic gas, pain, abdominal bloating and distension, and diarrhea is **small intestinal bacterial overgrowth**, or **SIBO**. This condition, which can also cause fatigue and body aches, is caused by an overabundance of bacteria in the small intestine.

The **migrating motor complex (MMC)** is a large muscular peristaltic wave which occurs about every 90-120 minutes between meals. This "housekeeping" wave pushes all the contents of the small intestine toward the colon, keeping the intestinal bacteria from moving backward.

Typically, large populations of bacteria are seen in the colon, with smaller amounts in the small intestine. If the MMC does not work properly, bacteria can migrate from the colon to the small bowel. They rapidly multiply and compete for nutrients with the host—us!

Different types of bacteria have various effects.

- Some harmful bacteria damage the absorptive lining of the small intestine, preventing absorption of nutrients from food.

Severe damage to the intestinal absorptive surface can result in **steatorrhea** (fatty diarrhea), weight loss, and deficiencies of fat-soluble Vitamins A, D, E, and K, Vitamin B_{12}, and calcium. Protein may be malabsorbed as well, requiring extra supplementation.

- Other bacteria species may cause bile acid diarrhea.

- Still other bacteria may result in gas and bloating, rather than diarrhea, as fermentable carbohydrates are converted to short-chain fatty acids. This is the reaction treated with the FODMAP diet.

Risk Factors for SIBO

Conditions considered higher risk for SIBO include:

- Scleroderma
- Diabetes (due to intestinal neuropathy)
- Gastroparesis (slow stomach emptying)
- Hypochlorhydria (decreased acid production in the stomach, which may be caused by long-term use of acid-suppressant medications)
- Stomach surgeries which have a "blind loop" (such as Roux-en-Y gastrojejunostomy)
- Small-intestinal strictures
- Intestinal pseudo-obstruction or other motility disorders
- Intestinal surgeries which remove the ileocecal valve
- Celiac disease
- Crohn's disease (with or without a history of surgery)

- Compromised immune system
- Aging

SIBO and Chronic Diarrhea

One study demonstrated SIBO is common in those with chronic diarrhea. Intense testing ruled out other causes for diarrhea, such as inflammatory bowel disease, celiac disease, infections, and structural and metabolic processes. This study demonstrated SIBO was present in 33 percent of patients, versus zero percent of control subjects[61]. *If you have chronic diarrhea, and all tests conducted by your physicians have been negative, consider getting tested for SIBO.*

Bacterial Overgrowth Theory of IBS

In recent years, Dr. Mark Pimentel's book, *A New IBS Solution,* has drawn more attention to SIBO, in what he calls the "bacterial overgrowth theory of IBS." His research demonstrated a high prevalence of SIBO amongst IBS patients. He has had positive results in treating his IBS patients with antibiotics.

However, other scientific studies have been unable to replicate Dr. Pimentel's research. The relationship between SIBO and IBS remains under debate.

Diagnosis and Treatment of SIBO

SIBO is typically diagnosed by hydrogen breath testing (either glucose or lactulose) if the bacterial population in the small intestine is greater than 10^5-10^6 organisms per milliliter.

The primary treatment for SIBO is antibiotics such as neomycin, levofloxacin, ciprofloxacin, metronidazole, Xifaxan®, or a combination of two of these medications. Unfortunately, many times after the course of antibiotics is complete, SIBO symptoms return. Some patients require cycling of the antibiotics, going on and off of them on a regular basis.

Another treatment is a short course of antibiotics followed by a long course of probiotics. The use of probiotics is controversial with SIBO. Some health professionals recommend and promote use of probiotics, while others caution introducing beneficial bacteria into a digestive system which is already overgrown with harmful species.

The overall goals for treatment of SIBO are:

- Treat the underlying cause of SIBO, if possible
- Restore the balance of small intestinal bacteria
- Provide nutritional support while the digestive tract heals and becomes able to resume healthy absorption of nutrients

Nutrition for SIBO

Nutrition care for SIBO depends on the severity of the bacterial overgrowth. Mild SIBO may require minimal vitamin supplementation until the digestive tract is repaired and normal absorption is restored.

Severe malabsorption may necessitate aggressive replenishment of vitamins, minerals, carbohydrates, protein, and fat. A registered dietitian can work with you to create a detailed plan to meet your specific needs.

Case Study:

A college-age client was diagnosed with IBS. We met together, and she made numerous dietary changes, but continued to have severe gas, pain, and bloating. Her physician eventually ordered a hydrogen breath test, which was positive for SIBO. After going on a course of Xifaxan®, her IBS symptoms were greatly improved. However, she continued to monitor the FODMAPs in her diet, or her symptoms returned.

Running and Diarrhea

As an avid runner, many times I have been in the middle of a challenging run when the diarrhea cramps hit. I know where all the

> Diarrhea affects an estimated 30-50% of runners.

public bathrooms are on my routes. A few times, I have even been forced to make an unplanned porta-potty stop.

Why is Diarrhea Common in Runners?

- When you are running, blood flow to the intestinal tract is diverted to the muscles. Any food in your stomach and intestines is not getting digested. Fermentable carbohydrates (FODMAPs) become food for the colonic bacteria, causing gas, bloating, and diarrhea.

- Gels and shot blocks can pull water into the gut, causing osmotic diarrhea. They are high in osmolality. Osmotic diarrhea may be an even greater issue when blood flow to the gut is decreased during intense workouts.

- Intestinal hormones can stimulate transit time, particularly in women. Anything in your intestines will move through even faster than normal.

- Anxiety about an upcoming race, workout, or life change can also increase intestinal motility. (Chapter 7)

- Physical jostling of stomach and intestinal contents may be a contributory factor. An interesting study demonstrated that cyclists do not have as much diarrhea as runners.

- Dehydration can cause diarrhea. Conversely, diarrhea can cause dehydration. Many runners do not sufficiently replace fluids while running, which can be a contributing factor.

Furthermore, the severity of runner's diarrhea is dependent on the level of effort, level of conditioning, degree of dehydration, and individual nervous system response of the gut (those with IBS have increased gut sensitivity).

How to Avoid Runner's Diarrhea (a.k.a. Runner's Trots)

- Start a journal. Track what changes you have made and if they have improved symptoms. (Appendix A and B)

- Experiment with timing of eating before a run. Some people benefit from avoiding food one to two hours prior to running.

- Run during different times of the day. Some people find that diarrhea only affects them during certain times of the day.

- Eat small amounts of easily digestible carbohydrates (such as starches and dairy products, if you tolerate them) and low-fat

> Personal tip: I take two Imodium® on race days or before long runs.

protein prior to a run. Examples include peanut butter and crackers, low-fat yogurt, a small bowl of low-fiber cereal with skim milk, low-fat cheese or cottage cheese with fruit, smoothie or shake, a banana, half a protein bar, and half a lunchmeat sandwich with very little else on it.

- If unsure which foods are aggravating your diarrhea, try the FODMAP elimination diet. (Chapter 10)

- Test different gels and blocks to see if you tolerate some better than others. (Many runners say Honey Stinger® energy gels are the most gut-friendly.) Always take them with plenty of water. A huge glob of concentrated sugar hitting your gut while you are running is likely to cause diarrhea.

- Moderate your intake of coffee, tea, energy drinks, and performance gels that include caffeine, which worsens diarrhea.

- Drink plenty of fluids, including water and electrolyte beverages.

- Get plenty of sleep. Personally, my gut always reacts poorly to a run when I haven't slept well the night before.

- Listen to your body. If you feel like you are going to have diarrhea before leaving the house to go for a run, don't ignore it! Better to stay home and wait until your tummy settles down than have to make an emergency pit stop.

Exercise-Induced Ischemic Colitis

Exercise-induced ischemic colitis (EIIC) is a type of diarrhea occurring in high-intensity endurance runners. The difference between runner's diarrhea and EIIC is that the diarrhea is mixed with bright red blood. Some people report that the severity of the cramping and diarrhea forces them to stop to use the bathroom during a run. Others report little cramping but have bloody diarrhea occurring immediately after an intense race or training run.

What Causes EIIC?

During strenuous exercise, blood flow to the intestinal tract may decrease by 80 percent.[70] Dehydration may also contribute to EIIC; if your body is low in fluids, this further decreases intestinal blood flow. Inadequate blood supply to the intestine means the tissue is not getting enough oxygen; it's like having a "stroke" in your colon. Without oxygen, small areas in the intestine may develop ulcers, or holes, which can bleed.

Other contributing causes of EIIC may include high body temperature (during running), use of oral contraceptives, or non-steroidal anti-inflammatory drugs (NSAIDs), such as ibuprofen, naproxen, and aspirin.

Treatment for EIIC

Though relatively uncommon, EIIC should be taken seriously. Unfortunately, the literature does not prescribe a standard treatment. Typically, this condition is treated with fluids, rest, avoiding NSAIDs and oral contraceptives, and reducing the intensity of training or competition. These strategies allow the bowel to heal on its own.

According to those who have personally experienced this frustrating condition, adequate hydration pre and post-race is a key component in managing EIIC. Unfortunately, loperamide (Imodium®) will not likely slow down the bowels enough to prevent symptoms of EIIC. Diet may play a role in managing this condition; use the guidelines offered for runner's diarrhea in the previous section.

If you experience symptoms of EIIC, please see your physician for evaluation, particularly if your symptoms include severe abdominal pain, vomiting, or excessive diarrhea. There have been rare cases where surgery was required to remove portions of damaged intestine.

Gas

As with diarrhea, gas is not a topic most people feel comfortable discussing. It may make you feel better knowing the average person produces one to three pints (0.5-1.7 liters) of gas daily, passing it about 14-23 times per day. For many, the main issue with gas is not how often it is passes, but the pain, bloating, and discomfort that accompany it.

People process foods differently. A food may cause gas for one person, while someone else enjoys the same food without problems. There are certain foods, drinks, and habits which can worsen symptoms. Gas is a by-product of chemical reactions in your gut. For example, gas from:

- beans and certain vegetables comes from *raffinose*

- dairy comes from *lactose*

- certain fruits comes from *fructose* and *sorbitol*

- wheat comes from *soluble fiber* and *fructans*

- some artificial sweeteners comes from *sorbitol*

Foods and Beverages Known to Cause Gas		
onions	turnips	apple juice
cabbage	parsnips	beer
peas	radishes	red wine
cucumbers	green peppers	carbonated beverages
potatoes	melons	milk and dairy products
Brussels sprouts	apples	eggs
cauliflower	peaches	bran and soluble fiber
broccoli	pears	wheat
sauerkraut	asparagus	corn
prunes	soy	gum and candy
dried fruit	lentils	containing sorbitol
beans (legumes)	nuts	

When eating and drinking, it is natural to swallow small amounts of air, which travels through the full length of the digestive tract, causing gas. If you are also eating gas-producing foods, it might be more than your gut can handle.

Below are some habits that cause us to swallow excess air and produce intestinal gas:

- Chewing gum and eating hard candy
- Smoking
- Drinking through a straw
- Skipping meals
- Mouth breathing
- Talking while eating
- Gulping food or beverages quickly

Strategies to Decrease Gas

Managing FODMAPs

You may have noticed many of the foods listed in the previous table were also mentioned earlier in the FODMAP diet. Following a low-FODMAP diet is one way of controlling excess gas. Not all types of fermentable carbohydrates will aggravate *your* symptoms. However, remember FODMAPs have a cumulative effect. The more FODMAPs you eat in one day, the more symptoms you are likely to feel. For example, you may be able to eat a few beans in a side salad at lunch, but if you pair the same salad with a glass of milk (lactose) and an apple (fructose and sorbitol), you may be in for an afternoon of misery.

Beano®

Beano® is an enzyme taken with beans to decrease gas. Unfortunately, Beano only works for foods containing the carbohydrate raffinose. Vegetables containing *raffinose* include asparagus, beans, broccoli, Brussels sprouts, cabbage, and cauliflower.

Lactaid®

Lactaid® tablets are digestive enzymes taken to help digest *lactose*, a carbohydrate found in dairy products. If your symptoms are from lactose maldigestion, taking lactase enzymes such as Lactaid® can improve gas and diarrhea. (Chapter 4)

Medications for Gas

There are numerous anti-gas medications on the market, including Maalox® Anti-Gas, Mylanta® Gas, Gas-X®, Phazyme®, and generic simethicone. Although widely used, their effectiveness is questionable. A gastroenterologist I know used to say, "Gas medications just turn thousands of tiny gas bubbles into one big one."

The Bottom Line

Hormones, excess bile acids, cancer treatments, small intestinal bacterial overgrowth, even running can adversely affect a sensitive GI tract. Gas, while completely normal, can be physically painful and socially ostracizing. There are many ways in which altering what we eat can decrease symptoms of gas, bloating, and diarrhea.

Chapter 17

Dehydration, Electrolytes, Vitamins, and Minerals

My patients with chronic diarrhea often complain of fatigue and exhaustion. In my experience, this is often due to dehydration, or inadequate water and electrolytes in the body.

Mechanism of Diarrhea and Dehydration

When you have diarrhea, your body loses extra water, plus the important electrolytes:

- Sodium
- Potassium
- Chloride

Those with inflammatory diarrhea (e.g. Crohn's disease, ulcerative colitis) or secretory diarrhea (e.g. carcinoid syndrome, Clostridium difficile) may have extreme losses of fluid and electrolytes, leading to a dangerous form of dehydration that can be life threatening.

Sodium

Sodium is plentiful in the foods that we eat—and combined with chloride—in the form of salt. Salt is added to processed, canned, frozen, and fast foods to extend shelf life and improve taste. While uncommon, those with chronic diarrhea can be at risk for **hyponatremia**, or low blood levels of sodium, due to extra losses from the stool.

Symptoms of low blood sodium include:

- loss of energy
- fatigue
- muscle weakness or cramps
- confusion
- nausea and vomiting
- headache

Potassium

Potassium is important for muscle and nerve cells. Low potassium in the blood, called **hypokalemia**, can be life-threatening. Severe hypokalemia often requires hospitalization and intravenous (IV) replacement.

High amounts of diarrhea may cause blood levels of potassium to drop too low. Symptoms of hypokalemia include:

- heartbeat irregularities
- fatigue
- muscle spasms or weakness

If you ever have any of the symptoms for low sodium or potassium, please contact your medical provider immediately.

Replacing Electrolytes

If you have chronic diarrhea, ensuring the diet includes adequate amounts of sodium and potassium is fairly simple. As previously mentioned, sodium is easy to find in food. Salty crackers and soups are favorite sodium replacements for many of my patients. Replacing potassium is a little trickier. Foods that contain high amounts of potassium include spinach, potatoes, tomatoes, citrus fruits, melons, bananas, dairy products, dried peas and beans, nuts, and chocolate. However, many of these foods are not tolerated by those with intestinal problems, so electrolyte beverages and replacements may be a better alternative.

Sports Drinks

Many people with chronic diarrhea treat their dehydration with sports drinks such as Gatorade®. Sports drinks are formulated to replace electrolytes lost in sweat during exercise. The quantities of sodium and potassium are not high enough to replace those lost by chronic diarrhea. Nevertheless, sports drinks may work for those with mild diarrhea, or if you are unable to access a better alternative.

Oral Rehydration Solutions (ORS)

Oral rehydration solutions (ORS) are beverages formulated especially for diarrhea. The World Health Organization (WHO) has studied and used oral rehydration solutions extensively in Third World countries for many years to treat severe diarrhea such as colera. In developing countries, untreated diarrhea in children, elderly, and the immune-compromised can be life-threatening.

> When traveling abroad, we bring ORS packets. They can be used for both traveler's and chronic diarrhea.

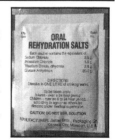

WHO developed a formula for oral rehydration salts that is relatively inexpensive to produce and distribute. This oral powder comes in individual packets that dissolve in one liter of clean drinking water.

You can make your own ORS at home with the following recipe:

> ### Homemade Oral Rehydration Solution
>
> - 2 level Tablespoons (TBSP) of sugar
> - ½ level teaspoon (tsp) of salt (sodium chloride)
> - ½ level teaspoon (tsp) of salt substitute (potassium chloride)
> - ½ level teaspoon (tsp) of baking soda, dissolved into
> - 4¼ cups (1 liter) of clean water
>
> You can also add sugar-free Crystal Light (I prefer lemonade flavor) or other sugar-free powdered beverage mix to improve taste.

Comparing Different Oral Rehydration Solutions

One of the difficulties in assessing ORS is identifying the quantities of sodium and potassium in a given volume. Sports drinks commonly list sodium and potassium in milligrams, whereas medical solutions list milliequivalents (mEq) per liter of solution. A conversion is required to convert mEq to milligrams.

The goal is to keep rehydration solutions as close as possible to a normal plasma osmolality of 285-295 milli-osmoles per kilogram, in order to maximize absorption and prevent osmotic diarrhea. (Chapter 4) Do not worry about the exact number. It is more important to realize the *higher the osmolality, the greater the chance of osmotic diarrhea.*

Oral Rehydration Solutions (ORS)

Drink	mg Na+ per 8oz.	mg K+ per 8oz.	Contains Carbs?	Osmolality* mOsm/kg
WHO ORS packets	413 mg	188 mg	Yes	245
Homemade ORS	414 mg	~300 (depends on salt substitute used)	Yes	~320
CeraLyte® 50	275 mg	188 mg	Yes	<225
CeraLyte® 70	386 mg	188 mg	Yes	<235
CeraLyte® 90	496 mg	188 mg	Yes	<260
Pedialyte®	244 mg	184 mg	Yes	250-270
Gatorade®	110-120 mg	30-45 mg	Yes	365
Propel®Zero	80 mg	20 mg	No	unknown
Clif Shot® electrolyte drink	180-200 mg	50 mg	Yes	unknown
NUUN Active Hydration Tablets	180 mg (per ½ tablet, dissolved in 8 oz water)	50 mg (per ½ tablet, dissolved in 8 oz water)	No	Unknown, but per the NUUN website, this product is hypotonic, or <285

*Normal plasma osmolality is 285-295 milli-osmoles per kilogram

Treating Dehydration with ORS

Something you may notice about both oral rehydration solutions and most sports drinks is that they both contain some form of sugar, usually in the form of glucose. When glucose is present, sodium and potassium absorption is increased. Therefore, rehydration beverages containing all three components—*sodium*, *potassium* and *glucose*—are recommended.

> Studies have shown glucose solutions less than 6% are not well absorbed by the intestine, whereas glucose solutions greater than 8% tend to cause GI distress.

When I recommend electrolyte replacement, it depends on the frequency and severity of the diarrhea. If one of my clients with chronic diarrhea complains about ongoing fatigue and severe diarrhea (15-25 trips to the bathroom each day), I recommend aggressive replacement of fluid and electrolytes with an ORS.

People with three or four stools per day may be able to use sports drinks or electrolyte-enhanced water, supplementing with ORS as needed.

How Much Fluid Do I Need Each Day?

It's best to try to exceed the established standard for **adequate intake (AI)**, especially if you have chronic diarrhea. Remember that all non-alcoholic, caffeinated-free fluids count toward your total, including water, ORS, juices, milk, herbal teas, decaf coffee, and soup. Even fruits and vegetables can contribute to your total fluid intake.

According to the Institute of Medicine, an adequate intake for...

- Men is about 3 liters (about 13 cups) of total fluids per day
- Women is 2.2 liters (about 9 cups) of total fluids per day

These guidelines do not take into account fluids lost during...

- Excessive sweating, which occurs in hotter climates and during summer months
- Exercise
- Diarrhea
- Breastfeeding

Tips for Getting Enough Fluid Each Day:

- Drink a beverage with each meal, then between meals too.

- Use a large water bottle labeled with ounces or liters to keep track of how much you are actually drinking. Take it everywhere you go.

- Don't forget to drink before, during, and after exercise.

- If you do not like the taste of plain water, try adding slices of lemon or lime to improve the flavor. Or, try non-caloric beverages such as Crystal Light® as tolerated.

- If you have diarrhea, room temperature water is often easier to tolerate than very cold water, which can cause cramping.

- Monitor the color of your urine. If it is very odorous and dark yellow, you are not drinking enough!

Vitamins and Minerals

Before launching into this topic, I will mention that, as a general rule, I am not a dietitian who advocates taking a lot of unnecessary supplements, especially vitamins and minerals. However, with gastrointestinal diseases and disorders, there are often particular vitamins and minerals which need supplementation. The following are examples, though your individual needs will vary.

Zinc

Zinc is a fascinating mineral. It supports immune function, helps proteins and hormones function properly, and is also part of the enzyme maintaining your sense of taste and smell.

If you have a lot of diarrhea, your body can get low in zinc. On the other hand, if you are low in zinc, it can cause diarrhea! Symptoms of low zinc levels include:

- Loss of taste or smell
- Hair loss
- Poor wound healing
- Decreased immune function
- Night blindness
- Infection
- Fatigue
- Diarrhea

Zinc status is hard to assess from laboratory tests, since blood tests do not accurately measure the total body levels. You can have normal blood tests for zinc and still be clinically deficient! Most doctors base the need for zinc supplementation on medical history and symptoms alone.

You have to be cautious when taking zinc supplements. They can cause nausea for some people, especially if taken on an empty stomach. Or, if you take too much zinc at once, it can actually *cause* diarrhea. Tricky balance!

Food sources of zinc: raw oysters, fortified breakfast cereal, beef, crab, baked beans, chicken

---

Recommended Dietary Allowances (RDAs) for Zinc:
- Men (>19 years old): 11 mg per day
- Women (>19 years old, not pregnant or lactating): 8 mg per day

---

Additional tips on zinc:

- Phytates (found in nuts and seeds) can bind to the zinc in your food, reducing your body's ability to absorb zinc.
- Zinc from animal products is more efficiently absorbed.
- Many cold lozenges contain zinc.

If a zinc supplement is needed:

- Zinc Sulfate 220 mg (discuss daily dose with MD or pharmacist).

Magnesium

Magnesium is important in supporting immune function, normal muscle and nerve function, bone structure, maintaining normal heart rhythms and blood pressure,

> Magnesium plays a role in over 300 metabolic functions in the body.

and regulating blood sugar levels. A physician will obtain a blood test to look for low magnesium, called hypomagnesemia.

Magnesium is absorbed in the ileum, the last portion of the small intestine. If the ileum is not functioning or has been resected (as with Crohn's disease), magnesium absorption may be compromised. Initially, low magnesium can result in symptoms of:

- Loss of appetite
- Nausea and/or vomiting
- Fatigue
- Weakness

Persistent low levels of magnesium can progress to:

- Numbness and tingling
- Muscle contractions and cramps
- Abnormal heart rhythms

Food sources of magnesium: whole grains, cereals, legumes, nuts, dark-green leafy vegetables (such as spinach), cocoa, tea, coffee

> **Recommended Dietary Allowances (RDAs) for magnesium:**
> - Men (19-30 years old): 400 mg per day
> - Men (>31 years old): 420 mg per day
> - Women (19-30 years old, not pregnant or lactating): 310 mg per day
> - Women (>31 years old, not pregnant or lactating): 320 mg per day

If a magnesium supplement is needed:

- Slow-Mag® (magnesium chloride) is absorbed more slowly and may cause less diarrhea.

- If your magnesium supplement causes or aggravates your diarrhea, discuss other options with your doctor or pharmacist.

- Avoid Milk of Magnesia (MOM), which is used to treat constipation.

- Avoid taking zinc supplements with magnesium, since zinc interferes with magnesium absorption.

- Some patients may require intravenous (IV) magnesium sulfate to bring blood levels up to normal range.

Vitamin B_{12}

Vitamin B_{12}, also called cobalamin, plays an important metabolic role in every cell of the body, is involved in DNA synthesis, and prevents **megaloblastic anemia**.

The lower half of the stomach produces an important protein called **intrinsic factor**. In the first part of the small intestine, Vitamin B_{12} and intrinsic factor bind together. When this pairing arrives in the ileum, they are absorbed together. If the stomach has been removed or bypassed, intrinsic factor will not be produced. As a result, very little Vitamin B_{12} can be absorbed from food. Likewise, without the ileum, the Vitamin B_{12} /intrinsic factor complex will pass through without getting absorbed.

Your body has several years of Vitamin B_{12} stores built up; however, you can become deficient once the reserve is depleted. If Vitamin B_{12} is not replaced before the stores are empty, irreversible peripheral nerve damage can occur. Low Vitamin B_{12} can result in symptoms of:

- Tiredness
- Weakness
- Weight loss
- Numbness and tingling in hands and feet
- Poor appetite
- Depression
- Problems with balance
- Confusion or dementia

Food sources of Vitamin B_{12}: beef, liver, clams, fish, poultry, eggs, milk & milk products, some fortified breakfast cereals

Dietary Reference Intakes (DRIs) for Vitamin B_{12}:
- Adults: 2.4 micrograms (mcg) per day

If Vitamin B_{12} levels are low and supplementation is required, there are several choices. Any of these three forms can deliver the Vitamin B_{12} your body needs.

- *Daily sublingual (under-the-tongue) tablets*—the body gets some passive absorption, meaning that if you take a concentrated dose of Vitamin B_{12}, some of it will cross the intestinal wall into the body.

- *Nascobal®, a Vitamin B$_{12}$ nasal spray* taken in one nostril once a week. It is absorbed directly from the nose into the bloodstream.

- *Monthly Vitamin B$_{12}$ intramuscular injections* — usually the cheapest, most commonly-used method of replacement.

Calcium

Ninety-nine percent of the total body calcium is stored in the bones and teeth. The small, yet important, one percent of body calcium is responsible for:

- Muscle function
- Nerve transmission
- Hormone secretion
- Sending signals within the cells
- Narrowing and dilation of blood vessels

Unfortunately, there are not very many obvious signs of calcium deficiency. Your body will even "steal" calcium from the bones to maintain body functions and keep blood levels within a very narrow range. When the body is deprived of adequate calcium for long periods of time, you may develop **osteopenia** or decreased bone *density*, and eventually **osteoporosis** which is decreased bone *mass*.

Those who have celiac disease, Crohn's disease, or history of a gastric bypass are at higher risk for malabsorption of calcium. This can be due to damage or surgical bypassing of the duodenum, the primary site of absorption for calcium. Also, many people with gastrointestinal problems avoid dairy products, which contain the highest proportion of calcium in the diet.

Food sources of calcium: dairy products (such as milk, yogurt and cheese), fish with bones (canned salmon and sardines), leafy green vegetables (spinach, kale, collard greens, broccoli), fortified orange juice

---

Dietary Reference Intakes (DRIs) for Calcium:

- Males (19-50 years) 1000 mg per day
- Males (>51 years)   1200 mg per day
- Females (19-50 years, including pregnant and lactating women) 1000 mg per day
- Females (>51 years) 1200 mg per day

Additional tips on calcium:

- Look at the nutrition label on the supplement. It will tell you the number of milligrams (mg) of elemental calcium in the product.
- Phytates (found in nuts and seeds) and oxalates (in spinach and soy) can reduce absorption of calcium.
- Absorption of calcium is lower when Vitamin D intake is low.
- Absorption of calcium is highest when taking less than 500 mg at one time, so it is better to split your doses of calcium rather than taking all at once. Take a 500 or 600 mg tablet twice a day.

If a calcium supplement is needed:

- Calcium carbonate is inexpensive, convenient, and best-absorbed if taken with food. However, calcium carbonate tends to cause more gas, bloating, and constipation than calcium citrate (e.g. Tums® and Rolaids®).
- Calcium citrate is a better choice for people with malabsorption.

Vitamin D

Vitamin D is a fat-soluble vitamin with many important functions:

- Promotes calcium absorption, enables normal bone mineralization and maintenance.
- Is a component of hormones.
- Plays a role in the immune function and reduction of inflammation.

Unfortunately, Vitamin D is available naturally in only a few foods. Once in the body, this vitamin must undergo a process called hydroxylation *twice* to be converted to its active form, calcitriol.

Vitamin D is also called the "sunshine vitamin" because the body can make its own supply. With only 20-30 minutes of sun exposure, the body can produce adequate amounts of Vitamin D, as long as you are not wearing any sunscreen, and your face, arms, and legs are exposed. Those who live in the northern latitudes are unable to get enough sun exposure for many months of the year, so Vitamin D insufficiency or deficiency is very common.

Most of my gastrointestinal patients require Vitamin D supplementation, due to a combination of insufficient intake and/or absorption, and possible lack of sun exposure.

Food sources of Vitamin D: fatty fish (salmon, tuna, and mackerel), fish liver oils, fortified orange juice, yogurt, ice cream, milk

---

Dietary Reference Intakes (DRIs) for Vitamin D:
- Males and Females (19-70 years) 600 IUs per day
- Males and Females (>70 years) 800 IUs day

If a Vitamin D supplement is needed:

- Over-the-counter Vitamin D supplements are usually Vitamin D_3. Studies indicate in higher doses, this form is better-absorbed. A typical dose for Vitamin D is 1000-2000 IUs per day.

- If blood tests indicate your Vitamin D levels are extremely low, your doctor may prescribe very high doses of supplements to get your levels back up.

- Prescription Vitamin D is often in the form of Vitamin D_2.

Iron

Iron is a mineral involved in transporting oxygen throughout the body. In addition, iron is a vital component of many enzymes and proteins, and is part of all the cells in the body. Low iron results in iron-deficiency anemia.

Iron is absorbed in the upper small intestine. If there is damage to the tissue in that area, iron absorption can be affected. In addition, certain conditions (such as excessive menstrual flow), diseases (such as Crohn's disease and ulcerative colitis), and surgeries (such as gastric bypass or Whipple procedure) can cause blood loss that exceeds absorption of iron.

Iron-deficiency anemia causes symptoms of fatigue, shortness of breath, and decreased immunity. Please see your doctor for a blood test to evaluate your iron status.

Food sources of heme iron (more easily-absorbed): organ meats (liver, heart), oysters, clams, beef, poultry

Food sources of non-heme (less easily-absorbed) iron: leafy green vegetables (spinach), beans and legumes, some fortified cereals and grains, watercress, tofu

Dietary reference Intakes (DRIs) for Iron:
- Males (>18 years) 8 mg per day
- Females (19-50 years) 18 mg per day
- Females (>18 years, pregnant) 27 mg per day
- Females (>18 years, lactating) 9 mg per day
- Females (>51 years) 8 mg per day

If your physician prescribes supplemental iron for you, here are a few important nutrition facts:

- Good news, iron supplements are constipating.

- Iron in food comes in two forms: heme and non-heme iron.

- Heme iron comes from animal products and is more easily absorbed. Non-heme iron comes from plant sources and must be converted by the body to heme iron prior to absorption. Thus, usually less iron is absorbed from plant sources.

- Iron supplements may cause stomach upset and are better-tolerated if taken with food.

- Vitamin C increases iron absorption from non-heme food. Taking your iron supplement with a food or drink containing Vitamin C (such as orange juice) promotes absorption.

- Tannins (from tea) and phytates (from legumes and whole grains) decrease iron absorption.

- Calcium and iron fight for absorption. If you are taking an iron supplement, do not take it with a food or supplement containing calcium in the same meal, or the body will likely take the calcium but leave the iron.

If iron supplements are needed:

- Ferrous fumarate, ferrous sulfate, and ferrous gluconate are the best-absorbed.

- Iron supplements can sometimes cause nausea. Many of my patients tolerate Slo-Fe (ferrous sulfate) better than others.

Other Vitamins

People with celiac disease, inflammatory bowel disease, or other malabsorption syndromes are at risk for other vitamin deficiencies as well, including Vitamin B6, folate, niacin, and riboflavin. If you suspect you are low in any of these nutrients, please discuss with your physician. For those with chronic malabsorption and malnutrition, I recommend daily adult multivitamins, in a chewable or liquid form to maximize absorption.

The Bottom Line

Dehydration often leads to chronic fatigue, due to the losses of electrolytes and fluid. Those with high-volume or high-frequency diarrhea must be diligent about fluid and electrolyte replacement, using oral rehydration solutions as needed.

Malabsorption of nutrients results in low levels of certain vitamins and minerals. Supplementation may be necessary to meet needs for growth and maintenance of body tissues and functions. Your doctor may need to run specific blood tests to determine if additional vitamins and minerals are necessary.

Chapter 18

Acute Diarrhea

Inevitably, people with chronic diarrhea will also occasionally get short-term or acute diarrhea. This may be a case of food poisoning, viral gastroenteritis ("the vomiting and diarrhea flu"), or traveler's diarrhea. Generally, acute diarrhea will resolve on its own. However, the following lists instances when medical intervention for acute diarrhea is advised.

Medical Intervention Indicated for Acute Diarrhea

- Diarrhea in infants.

- Moderate or severe diarrhea in young children.

- Acute diarrhea for more than 72 hours.

- Diarrhea associated with blood.

- Diarrhea that continues for more than two weeks.

- Diarrhea that is associated with more general illness such as non-cramping abdominal pain, fever, weight loss, etc.

- Diarrhea in travelers (more likely to have exotic infections such as parasites).

- Diarrhea in food handlers (potential to infect others).

- Diarrhea in institutions (hospitals, child care, mental health institutes, geriatric and convalescent homes).

Traveler's Diarrhea Case Study:

After traveling to Costa Rica, my mom had diarrhea for several weeks. She finally called her primary care doctor, who said that by eating she was "feeding the bug." In order to "starve the bug," she was advised to drink only Gatorade for 24 hours and not to eat any food. She followed this advice, and the diarrhea went away. When she experienced traveler's diarrhea on subsequent vacations, she went back on the Gatorade-only diet, and within a few days, the diarrhea resolved itself.

Treatment for Acute Diarrhea

Acute diarrhea can quickly lead to dehydration, particularly in those who already suffer from chronic diarrhea. Mild-to-moderate dehydration is treated by drinking oral rehydration solutions (ORS) to replace what was lost through diarrhea or vomiting. (Chapter 17) Begin with small sips of ORS, such as one to two ounces every fifteen minutes, and increase the volume slowly as tolerated.

If acute diarrhea persists, it can lead to severe dehydration. Those with any of the following symptoms should seek medical attention immediately:

- Very dry skin— when pinched, stays in a "tented" position and does not snap back to normal
- Extreme thirst
- Confusion or delirium
- Irritability
- Very dry mouth

- Sunken eyes
- Lack of tears
- Lack of sweating
- Rapid breathing and heart rate
- Little or no urine output

The Bottom Line

The focus of treatment for acute diarrhea is treatment of dehydration. While mild or moderate dehydration can usually be treated at home, those with symptoms of severe dehydration should seek medical treatment immediately.

Chapter 19

Discussing Diarrhea with your Doctor

By the time you read this book, many or most of you will already have met with your primary care provider or a gastroenterologist. For those of you who have not, here is helpful information to bring when you visit a physician.

Information to Bring to Your Doctor

- General medical history, including any treatment for cancer.

Significant Weight Loss	Severe Weight Loss
5% in 1 month	>5% in 1 month
7.5% in 3 months	>7.5% in 3 months
10% in 6 months	>10% in 6 months
20% in 12 months	>20% in 12 months

- Surgical history. Please obtain a surgical report if possible, particularly if certain parts of your digestive system have been removed or re-routed.

- Weight history, especially if you have lost a significant amount of weight in less than six months.

- Previous diagnostic tests, such as endoscopy, colonoscopy, abdominal ultrasound, CT scans, or small bowel follow-through.

- Labs from the past two years.

- List of current prescribed medications, including any recent antibiotic use, as well as over-the-counter supplements and herbals.

- Pertinent social history, recent travel, and/or current emotional stressors.

- Family history of GI diseases and disorders.

- Food allergies or intolerances, and what your reaction is to each (i.e. wheezing, hives, diarrhea, vomiting, etc.). Also, how the allergy/intolerance was diagnosed, such as by an allergist, naturopath, blood test, skin prick, or self.

GI-Specific Questions

- How long ago did the diarrhea begin—weeks, months, or years?

- Was it gradual or acute?

- Have you lost weight?

- Did the diarrhea begin after travel to a foreign country?

- Do you have a fever?

- What is the frequency and timing of the diarrhea? Does it occur during the daytime only, at night only, or both day and night? Do you have diarrhea after certain meals?

- Is the diarrhea continuous or intermittent? Are there certain days of the week the diarrhea is better or worse?

- Does the diarrhea stop when you stop eating?

- Do you have pain? Is the pain relieved after a bowel movement?

- Any nausea or vomiting?

- Heartburn, dyspepsia, or reflux?

- Problems swallowing?

- Can you describe the consistency of the diarrhea? Is it watery, bloody, frothy, or greasy (floating)?

- Is there undigested food in the stool?

- Are there foods you have noticed make the diarrhea better or worse?

- Are you taking medications that help the diarrhea?

- Do you feel weak and tired? Has the diarrhea affected your normal activities? How?

Food Journal

Keep a journal of your food intake and diarrhea output for a week before you go to the doctor. See Appendix A and B for sample journals. Bring the journal with you to the doctor's appointment.

Keeping food records can be cumbersome, but this information is extremely valuable for a doctor or dietitian. It helps them make connections between your dietary intake and chronic diarrhea.

GI Apps

If you do not like the idea of writing down this sensitive information, there are free apps for your smart phone too. Here are a few to try:

- GI Monitor
- MyGiTrack
- Bowel Mover Lite
- Crohn's Diary
- GI Buddy (from the Crohn's and Colitis Foundation of America)

The Bottom Line

Be prepared for your doctor's appointment. Bring all medical and gastrointestinal history information, a week's worth of food records, and any questions you want to ask the doctor. It will help the doctor formulate a plan of care specific for your needs.

Chapter 20

Nutritional Needs for Diarrhea

Registered dietitians use many clinical methods to make sure you are getting enough nutrition. We look at medical history, weight history, certain lab values, and even the visual appearance of the person sitting in front of us.

If you have lost a significant amount of weight unintentionally, you need to discuss this with your primary care provider. Weight loss can be a symptom of a more serious illness or disorder.

Estimating Nutrition Needs

Dietitians have several ways to estimate calorie and protein needs. Here is one way to estimate your nutrition needs on your own. However, keep in mind that these are basic calculations; your particular needs may be different, based on your history and diagnosis.

Converting Weight from Pounds to Kilograms

- Weight in pounds (lbs) divided by 2.2 = Weight in kilograms (kg)

Calculating Calories Needed Per Day

- Weight in kg x 20 calories per kg = calories to help you *lose* weight

- Weight in kg x 25 calories per kg = calories to *maintain* weight
- Weight in kg x 30 calories per kg = calories to help you *gain* weight
- Weight in kg x 35 calories per kg = calories for *severe malabsorption or illness*

Calculating Protein Needs Per Day

- Weight in kg x 0.8 grams per kg = grams of protein needed for *basic body functions* and maintenance
- Weight in kg x 1.2 grams per kg = grams of protein needed for *chronic diarrhea* losses
- Weight in kg x 1.2-1.5 grams per kg = grams of protein needed *after surgery*
- Weight in kg x 1.5-1.8 grams per kg = grams of protein needed to replace protein stores *for IBD flare, chronic malabsorption, short bowel syndrome, or after acute illness*

The Bottom Line

If you are losing weight, you likely need more calories and protein. You may also need additional vitamin supplementation. A registered dietitian can personalize a meal plan to meet your specific needs.

Conclusion

My first goal is to *provide you* with tools and knowledge. My second goal is to *empower you* to find different solutions to find out what works *for you*. Remember, we are all different; one size does not fit all. Life is a marathon, not a sprint. Pace yourself. You can do it!

Thank you for taking this journey with me. I would love to hear your personal success stories!

Niki Strealy, RD, LD
The Diarrhea Dietitian
niki@diarrheadietitian.com

Glossary of Terms

Absorption—the uptake of nutrients into the body.

Active transport—movement of electrolytes, glucose, and amino acids across a cell membrane against the concentration gradient from low to high; this requires energy from the cells.

Allergen—antigens which cause an allergic response from the immune system.

Anaphylaxis—a very rapid, serious allergic reaction which can be life-threatening. It is a hypersensitivity to foreign proteins or medications resulting from sensitization following prior contact with the causative agent. Symptoms include rash, tongue and throat swelling, and low blood pressure.

Antibody—a protein produced by the immune system after coming in contact with proteins (antigens) identified by the immune system as harmful invaders. It can also be produced when the immune system responds inappropriately to benign substances such as protein from food (e.g. gluten; casein). Is a type of immunoglobulin.

Antibiotic-associated diarrhea (AAD)—frequent, watery diarrhea occurring after treatment with antibiotics used to treat bacterial infections.

Antigen—an environmental substance, including viruses, bacteria, pollen, chemicals, and food proteins, which causes the immune system to create antibodies against it. The antigen and antibody fit together like a lock and key.

Bile acid malabsorption or **Chronic idiopathic bile acid diarrhea**— a condition where excess bile is produced by the liver, causing bile salt diarrhea.

Bolus—a ball-shaped mass moving through the digestive tract, especially from mouth to stomach.

Bowel obstruction—a blockage of either the small or large intestine which prevents food from moving through the digestive tract. It can spontaneously resolve or require surgical removal.

Brush border—microvilli on the surface of the intestinal villi which expand the surface area and assist with absorption of carbohydrates such as lactose. Looks similar to the bristles on a paintbrush.

Carbohydrates—the body's most important source of energy. The digestive system breaks down carbohydrates into glucose, then uses this glucose (blood sugar) as energy for cells, tissues and organs. Extra carbohydrates are stored in the liver and muscles for later use.

Carcinoid syndrome—a collection of symptoms caused by tumors which secrete a vasoactive substance called serotonin. Symptoms include flushing, nausea, vomiting, secretory diarrhea, and shortness of breath. Treatment includes surgery to remove tumors and management of serotonin through medications. Suggested diet changes include avoiding foods with tyramine and increasing intake of foods containing tryptophan.

Celiac disease—an inherited, autoimmune disease which causes flattening of intestinal villi when exposed to gluten, which is contained in wheat, rye, barley, and their derivatives. Its only treatment is a 100 percent gluten-free diet.

Chyme—the semi-fluid mass of partly digested food once it has exited the stomach into the duodenum.

Clostridium difficile, also known as C. diff—a bacterium which causes severe secretory diarrhea, and can result in life-threatening toxic megacolon.

Colectomy—removal of all (total) or part (hemi-) of the colon.

Colon or **large intestine**—the last section of the digestive system. Its function is to remove water and salt from liquid waste, forming a mass called stool.

Colostomy—a surgical procedure whereby the colon is pulled out to the surface of to the skin and an opening is created. Bowel movements leave the body through the opening into a pouch attached to the skin.

Denaturation—the process whereby the bonds between amino acids (proteins) begin to break down in the stomach in preparation for absorption in the small intestine.

Diagnosis of exclusion—a medical diagnosis reached by a process of elimination, rather than direct identification through blood work, procedures, biopsies, or examination.

Dietary fructose intolerance or **fructose malabsorption (FM)**—a condition where the body cannot digest the sugar fructose, resulting in gas, bloating, and osmotic diarrhea. It is commonly associated with **irritable bowel syndrome** and diagnosed with hydrogen breath testing. Treatment involves reducing fructose intake or avoiding foods—especially fruits—with a high fructose-to-glucose ratio.

Digestion—the process of breaking down food into a simpler form, so it can be absorbed and used by the body.

Dumping syndrome or rapid gastric emptying—a condition where ingested foods bypass the stomach too rapidly and enter the small intestine largely undigested. These hypertonic stomach contents in the small intestine can cause water to be pulled rapidly into the intestinal lumen, resulting in osmotic diarrhea. "Early" dumping begins within one-half to one hour after a meal; symptoms include nausea, vomiting, cramping, bloating, diarrhea, dizziness, and fatigue. "Late" dumping occurs one to three hours after eating; symptoms include weakness, sweating, and dizziness.

Duodenum—the first and shortest portion of the small intestine, where chemical digestion begins. It is the site of absorption for calcium and iron.

Dysbiosis—an imbalance of microorganisms in the body, especially in the digestive tract or on the skin. It is often associated with digestive and autoimmune disorders, such as **inflammatory bowel disease**, chronic fatigue syndrome, and **irritable bowel syndrome**. Symptoms include fatigue, gas, bloating, diarrhea, and constipation.

Enterochromaffin cells—a particular type of cell lining the respiratory tract and digestive system which secretes approximately 90 percent of the body's **serotonin**.

Enzymes—a chain of amino acids which chemically breaks down macronutrients into simpler forms so they can be used by the body.

Esophageal sphincter (lower)—a muscular valve separating the esophagus from the stomach. It allows the food bolus to pass into the stomach while preventing stomach acid from regurgitating back up into the esophagus.

Esophagogastrectomy—the surgical removal of the lower portion of the esophagus and upper part of the stomach, usually due to esophageal cancer.

Exercise-induced ischemic colitis (EIIC)—a condition which can occur after long strenuous exercise, caused by compromised blood flow to the colon, resulting in bloody diarrhea.

Fats—a source of energy for the body. They also help with the absorption of fat-soluble vitamins A, D, E and K, and provide cushioning to the internal organs.

Flare—a period of active disease or recurrence of symptoms for those with a chronic condition, such as Crohn's disease or ulcerative colitis.

Food allergy—a rejection of a food or substance by the immune system. Symptoms occur in many organs, and can include hives, rash, itching, wheezing, swelling of eyelids, lips, mouth, tongue and throat, nasal congestion, abdominal pain, vomiting, diarrhea, and low blood pressure.

Food intolerance—the body's inability to process a particular food or additive which does not involve activation of the immune system.

Food sensitivity—a term used when it is unclear if a reaction is due to a food allergy or intolerance.

Functional food— foods which include an extra ingredient that can exert a positive health effect beyond basic nutrition. Examples include soluble fiber in oatmeal or calcium-fortified orange juice.

Gastrectomy—a partial (subtotal) or full (total) surgical removal of the stomach.

Gastrocolic reflex—an increase in peristalsis after eating a meal which causes the urge to have a bowel movement.

Gastroesophageal reflux disease (GERD) —a chronic condition caused by acid refluxing up from the stomach into the esophagus. Symptoms include heartburn and nausea. GERD can cause mucosal damage from the stomach acid. Treatment usually includes medication and dietary modification.

Gastroenterologist—a physician specializing in treating the diseases and disorders affecting the gastrointestinal tract and accessory organs, including the liver, gallbladder, and pancreas.

Gluten—a protein found in wheat and related grain species barley and rye. The body's reaction to this protein is the cause of **celiac disease**.

Glycoprotein—an important membrane protein which plays a role in cell-to-cell interactions; see **intrinsic factor**.

Hydrogen breath test—a test to evaluate for lactose intolerance fructose intolerance, and SIBO. It is best conducted in a medical facility to assure accuracy.

Hydrolyze—to break chemical bonds by adding water. For example, lactose is hydrolyzed into its monosaccharide components, glucose and galactose, to allow for absorption in the small intestine.

Hyperosmolar/Hyperosmolality—abnormally increased osmolar concentration in relation to normal body fluids. See **osmolality**.

Hypokalemia—low levels of potassium in the blood; normal blood potassium is 3.5-5.0 mEq/L.

Hyponatremia—low levels of sodium in the blood; normal blood sodium is 135-145 mEq/L. Sodium blood levels below 125 mEq/L are severe hyponatremia.

Ileostomy—a surgical procedure where the ileum is pulled out to the surface of to the skin and an opening is created. Liquid bowel movements leave the body through the opening into a pouch attached to the skin.

Ileum—the third portion of the small intestine, after the duodenum and the jejunum, ending at the ileocecal valve, which opens into the large intestine. It is the main site of absorption for Vitamin B_{12} and magnesium, and it contains large numbers of immune system cells.

Immunoglobulin (Ig) — a glycoprotein which functions as an antibody. There are five classes or subtypes, IgA, IgD, IgE, IgG, and IgM.

Immunoglobulin E (IgE) — the antibody associated with type 1 hypersensitivity reactions such as anaphylaxis.

Inflammatory bowel disease (IBD — a group of inflammatory conditions and diseases of the small and large bowel; the most common types are Crohn's disease and ulcerative colitis.

Intestinal permeability — see **leaky gut syndrome.**

Intrinsic factor — a glycoprotein produced by the cells in the fundus of the stomach, which is necessary for the absorption of Vitamin B_{12} in the ileum.

Iron-deficiency anemia — a type of anemia caused by poor dietary intake or malabsorption of iron, or from iron loss caused by bleeding.

Irritable bowel syndrome (IBS) — a chronic functional disorder of the intestinal tract, characterized by constipation and/or diarrhea, cramping abdominal pain, and the passage of mucus in the stool.

Isotonic — liquids with equal osmotic pressure or same concentration; normal plasma osmolarity is 275-295 mOsm/Liter.

Jejunum — the middle section of the small intestine, containing both circular and longitudinal muscles, which aids in peristalsis. It is a major site of both carbohydrate and protein absorption.

J-pouch — a surgically-created internal pouch which serves as a holding reservoir for stool, similar to a rectum, for people who have had the entire colon removed, and who do not have an ileostomy.

Lactase — an enzyme produced by the body which breaks the chemical bonds of lactose, allowing it to be absorbed.

Lactose — a type of carbohydrate (sugar) found in milk.

Lactose intolerance — a condition occurring when the body does not make enough lactase enzymes to break down lactose for absorption.

Large intestine — see **colon**

Leaky gut syndrome or **intestinal permeability**—while not accepted as a formal medical diagnosis, refers to a condition where the intestinal lining is damaged. This increases its permeability, allowing whole proteins, toxins, and other invaders into the bloodstream, which may affect the immune system.

Macronutrients— carbohydrates, fats, and protein, the building blocks of the human diet. They provide calories for energy, growth, and other body functions.

Malnutrition—a condition that occurs when the body does not get enough nutrients. It may be caused by inadequate or unbalanced diet, poor digestion or absorption, anorexia, or insufficient food intake.

Megaloblastic anemia—a condition where red blood cells are larger than normal. It can be caused by a deficiency of Vitamin B_{12} or folic acid.

Micronutrients—nutrients such as vitamins and minerals which are required by the human body in small quantities but cannot be produced by the body itself. They allow the body to produce enzymes, hormones, and other essential substances required for growth and development.

Migrating motor complex (MMC)—a specific pattern of peristaltic activity occurring in the smooth muscle of the esophagus, stomach and small intestine between meals. Called the "housekeeper" of the digestive system, it occurs about every 75-90 minutes between meals, lasts approximately 15 minutes, and is separated into four distinct phases, any of which can be halted if food enters the body. It is regulated by the central nervous system and the digestive hormone motilin, and is thought to prevent colonic bacteria from migrating backward into the small intestine.

Mucosa—the lining of the intestinal tract.

Non-celiac gluten sensitivity—a non-allergenic, non-autoimmune condition caused by an adverse reaction to gluten. Symptoms include abdominal pain, diarrhea, migraine, mental confusion, lethargy, and limb and muscular pain, appearing within hours or days of gluten exposure. Treatment is a 100 percent gluten-free diet.

Oral rehydration solution (ORS) or **oral rehydration therapy (ORT)**—a simple oral solution of electrolytes and sugars which is taken for dehydration associated with diarrhea, particularly severe secretory diarrhea, such as cholera or rotavirus.

Osmolality—the concentration of a solution in terms of osmoles of dissolved solute per kilogram of solvent. The normal range of serum osmolality is 285-295 mOsm/kg, which is considered isotonic.

Osteopenia—a condition where the density of bone mineral is lower than normal. It is considered a normal sign of aging but can also be a precursor to osteoporosis.

Osteoporosis—a condition where thinning of the bones leads to an increased risk of fractures. Risk factors include female gender, low weight, low sex hormones during menopause, smoking, history of poor calcium absorption or intake, and certain medications such as steroids.

Pancreatic enzymes—prescription medication containing enzymes to help digest fat, protein, and carbohydrates. It is taken with all meals and snacks for treatment of **pancreatic insufficiency**.

Pancreatic insufficiency—the lack of necessary digestive enzymes made by the pancreas, which leads to malabsorption of food. Symptoms include fatty diarrhea (**steatorrhea**), gas, abdominal pain, bloating, and weight loss.

Passive transport or absorption—movement of electrolytes, glucose, and amino acids across a cell membrane which requires no energy from the cells. There are four types: diffusion, facilitated diffusion, filtration, and osmosis.

Peristalsis—smooth muscle contractions which propel food and liquids through the digestive tract.

Prebiotics—indigestible fibers and sugars which support the growth and metabolic activity of probiotics.

Probiotics—organisms live in the intestinal tract and protect the host from disease.

Protein—a macronutrient consisting of one or more linked amino acids. Proteins are broken down into polypeptides, then peptides, and finally, amino acids, which can then be used to build, support, and maintain the body structure, repair tissues, and function as essential components of hormones and enzymes.

Pyloric sphincter or valve—a strong ring of smooth muscle separating the stomach from the duodenum. During digestion, it regulates the speed with which food and liquid leave the stomach.

Randomized controlled trials (RCT)—a scientific experiment which tests the effectiveness of various medications, foods, devices, surgery, methods, or treatments on the body; considered the "gold standard" of clinical trials. Study subjects are placed in separate, random groups, and neither the scientist nor the patient knows if the study subject will receive the prescribed treatment or a placebo. Variables are controlled as much as possible, to isolate the cause and effect relationship of the applied treatment.

Remission—a period of time without active disease for those with a chronic illness.

Saturated fat—the most harmful type of fat, it can increase the risk of both Type 2 diabetes and cardiovascular disease. It is found in animal products—whole milk dairy, lard, and fatty meats—as well as vegetable products—coconut, cottonseed, palm kernel oil, and cocoa butter (used in chocolate).

Secretion—the process of creating a substance, then releasing or oozing that substance from cells or bodily fluids. Examples: digestive enzymes, intrinsic factor.

Serotonin—a neurotransmitter created from the essential amino acid tryptophan, which is mainly found in the digestive system. Its main function is to regulate intestinal movements.

Short bowel syndrome (SBS)—a condition where the small intestine is either surgically removed or damaged to a point where it cannot absorb enough nutrients or fluid to maintain healthy body functions.

Small intestinal bacterial overgrowth (SIBO)—a condition of excessive bacterial growth in the small intestine. Symptoms include nausea, gas, bloating, and diarrhea. SIBO is typically treated with periodic cycling of antibiotics and/or a combination of antibiotics, probiotics, and dietary changes.

Steatorrhea—the presence of excess fat in bowel movements. Stools may also float in the toilet water, have an oily appearance, and be especially foul-smelling. It can result in significant weight loss, malabsorption of fat-soluble Vitamins A, D, and E, and Vitamin B_{12}.

Tight junctions or **zonula occludens**—cells sandwiched together so closely there is no intercellular space. Found in the digestive tract, they form an impermeable barrier to food and fluids.

Trans fats—created in the manufacturing process when unsaturated fats are partially hydrogenated. Trans fats increase the risk of cardiovascular disease.

Transdermal patch—a patch that delivers medication through the skin and into the bloodstream, it is commonly used for pain medications (such as Fentanyl) and estrogen.

Transit time—the amount of time it takes food to travel from mouth to anus.

Total parenteral nutrition (TPN) —an intravenous feeding method whereby the digestive tract is bypassed. Nutrition needs are met with a specific nutritional formula containing carbohydrates (as glucose), proteins (as amino acids) and fat (as lipids), in addition to vitamins, minerals, and other essential nutrients.

Tube Feeding—pre-made formulas which are fed through a tube directly into the digestive system. Feeding tubes may go through the nose and into the stomach or small intestine, or may be surgical placed directly into the stomach or small intestine.

Villi—tiny, finger-like projections that protrude from the lining of the small intestine;. They are connected to the bloodstream so nutrients can be quickly absorbed and distributed in the body. Villi increase the absorptive surface area of the digestive system, allowing more absorption of essential nutrients.

Whipple procedure or **pancreaticoduodenectomy**—a surgical operation which removes the bottom section of the stomach, first and second portions of the gall bladder, head of the pancreas, common bile duct, and the gallbladder, as a treatment for pancreatic tumors. A similar procedure involves preserving the stomach, while removing the other organs.

Appendix A
Daily Journal

Date: Day: This week, I am trying/avoiding:

Time	Food or Beverage	Serving Size	Activity/ Exercise	Symptoms	BM Type	Comments

GI Descriptions:
B-bloated
Con-constipated
Cr-crampy
G-gassy
N-normal/pretty good

BM Type (Bristol Stool Chart used by permission):
1-Hard lumps, like nuts
2-Sausage-shaped but lumpy
3-Like a sausage, but with cracks on its surface
4-Like a sausage, smooth and soft
5-Soft blobs with clear-cut edges
6-Fluffy pieces with ragged edges, mushy
7-Watery, no solid pieces

Appendix B
Daily Journal Sample

Date: 1/24/2013   Day: Thursday This week, I am trying/avoiding sorbitol

Time	Food or Beverage	Serving Size	Activity/ Exercise	Symptoms	BM Type	Comments
6:45am	Wake up			N		
7:30 AM	Life Cereal Skim milk Coffee NF creamer	¾ cup ½ cup 2 (8oz) cups 2 TBSP				
9 AM			Walked to bus stop (1/4 mile)	B, Cr	7	took 2 imodium
10AM	String cheese Saltine crackers	1 stick 4		Better tummy, but still cr		
12Pm	Subway sand w/ chicken, veggies, mayo, mustard Choc chip cookie Water	6 inch 1 16oz.				
2:30pm				B, C		
4pm	Apple	1 Golden delicious	Walk home from bus (¼ mi)		6	
6pm	Sliced ham Mashed potatoes Side salad- lettuce, tom, cucumbers, dressing Water	2 slices ½ cup ½ cup 2 TBSP 12 oz.				
8pm				B, Cr, G	6	
10:30 pm	Fish crackers	½ cup				
11:00 pm	Bed			N		

GI Descriptions:
- **B**-bloated
- **Con**-constipated
- **Cr**-crampy
- **G**-gassy
- **N**-normal/pretty good

BM Type (Bristol Stool Chart used by permission):
- **1**-Hard lumps, like nuts
- **2**-Sausage-shaped but lumpy
- **3**-Like a sausage, but with cracks on its surface
- **4**-Like a sausage, smooth and soft
- **5**-Soft blobs with clear-cut edges
- **6**-Fluffy pieces with ragged edges, mushy
- **7**-Watery, no solid pieces

Appendix C
Easy-To-Digest and Low-Fiber Diet

Food Group	Choose	Limit or Avoid
Meats and Proteins	Tender baked, boiled, broiled, barbequed, creamed or roasted beef, lamb, pork, poultry, veal, or fish; eggs; smooth tofu; smooth peanut butter	Dried peas, beans and lentils; *refried beans; legumes; nuts; meats with tough connective tissue; fried meats; meats with spicy seasoning; corned beef; lunch meat with nitrates; meats with casings such as sausage and hot dogs; chunky peanut butter
Breads, Cereals and Grains	Refined cooked cereal such as Cream of Wheat, oatmeal, and grits; Refined dry puffed wheat or rice cereal; sourdough or white bread; refined wheat or light rye bread; biscuits; plain bagels and muffins; plain soda and graham crackers; noodles, pasta and macaroni; white rice; plain pastries; pretzels; waffles and pancakes; cornmeal, used in corn chips or cornbread	Unrefined or bran cereals; granola; Grape Nuts; wheat germ; shredded wheat; whole grain breads or breads containing seeds, nuts, or dried fruit; whole grain or wild rice; fried or spicy breads and starches (i.e. jalapeno bread)
Vegetables and Vegetable Juices	All vegetable juices; canned or cooked tender asparagus tips, artichoke hearts, beets, green beans, carrots, onion, summer squash, zucchini and pumpkin; all potatoes without skin, including potato chips; other vegetables may be juiced if no pulp included	Whole or raw vegetables such as corn, celery, mushrooms, cabbage, peas, broccoli, bean sprouts, stir fry vegetables, sauerkraut, spinach, lima beans, sweet peppers; vegetables with skins and seeds; raw vegetables including lettuce; spicy vegetables such as chili peppers and jalapenos

Food Group	Choose	Limit or Avoid
Fruits and Fruit Juices	All fruit juices; canned fruit without skins and seeds, such as **applesauce**, pears, apricots, peaches, cherries, mandarin oranges, and fruit cocktail; **ripe bananas**; avocados	All other raw fruits and fruits with skins and seeds, such as berries; dried fruits including raisins, dates, figs, currants, and prunes
*Milk and Milk Products	Milk; **boiled milk**; cream; **cheese**; cottage cheese; yogurt- plain, custard-style, or with soft fruit; frozen yogurt; ice cream as tolerated	Yogurt with berries
Fats	Margarine; butter; cooking oil; cream and cream substitutes; mayonnaise; salad dressings	Spicy salad dressings or those with seeds; olives
Beverages	Milk; cocoa; juice; decaffeinated beverages	Caffeinated beverages; carbonated beverages or alcohol may cause gas and distention (these do not contain fiber, but may worsen diarrhea)
Desserts and Sweets	Those made with allowed foods including cakes, cookies, candy, custard, **gelatin**, ice cream, sherbet, sorbet, pies, puddings, and **tapioca**; **marshmallows**	Those containing nuts, seeds, *coconut, raisins, currants, or any other foods to avoid; chocolate (does not contain fiber, but can have a laxative effect)
Soups	Bouillon; broth; broth based and cream soups made with allowed foods	Soups containing lentils, legumes and any other foods to avoid
Miscellaneous	Salt; pepper; sugar; honey; jelly; syrup; mild mustard and ketchup; vanilla and other flavoring extracts; lemon juice; vinegar; soy sauce; white sauce and mild gravies; mild spices and herbs	*Coconut; popcorn; seeds; pickles; relish; spicy mustard; nuts; Tabasco or hot sauce; strong spices such as chili peppers, horseradish or curry powder; jam or Marmalade

Note: Foods highlighted in **bold** on the **Choose** list are "thickening" or constipating foods.

*These foods are tolerated by some people, but may aggravate diarrhea in others

Appendix D
Low–Lactose Diet

Food Group	Choose	Limit or Avoid
Meats and Proteins	Plain meat, poultry, or fish; Kosher hot dogs and luncheon meats; tofu and soy products; natural peanut butter; nuts and seeds; eggs	Cream sauces; cheese, cheese spreads, cottage cheese; omelets; quiche; soufflés prepared with milk or cheese; peanut butter with added milk solids
Breads, Cereals and Grains	Italian or French bread; graham crackers; saltine crackers; bagels; oatmeal, rice cereals, cream of wheat; rice, pasta or macaroni	Mixes- muffin, biscuit, waffle, pancake, and cake; macaroni and cheese; creamed, scalloped, or au gratin potatoes
Vegetables and Vegetable Juices	All vegetable juices and vegetables prepared without milk or dairy (such as cheese)	Creamed, breaded, or buttered vegetables
Fruits and Fruit Juices	All are allowed	None
Milk and Milk Products	Lactaid milk; soy milk, rice, almond or hemp milk; soy cheese or yogurt; lactose-free yogurt	Milk (including powdered); cream; cheese; cottage cheese; sour cream; yogurt; frozen yogurt; ice cream; cheese spreads
Fats	Margarine; cooking oil; shortening; non-dairy creamer and whipped toppings; mayonnaise; salad dressings; gravy made with water	Butter; cream; cream cheese; sour cream; milk-based dressings, sauces, and dips; whipped cream; gravy made with milk
Beverages	Non-dairy milk substitutes; carbonated drinks; fruit juices/drinks; lemonade; nutritional supplements such as Ensure or Boost	Milk (whole, lowfat, nonfat); half and half, cream; powdered, condensed, and evaporated milk; cocoa; goat, acidophilus, and chocolate milk; Ovaltine; instant breakfast

Food Group	Choose	Limit or Avoid
Desserts and Sweets	Non-dairy sorbet; frozen fruit bars; angel food cake; jello; honey; sugar; syrup; molasses; jam, jelly, preserves	Ice cream; sherbet; ice milk; frozen yogurt; chocolate and fudge; pudding, custard, cakes and pies made with milk; toffee; caramel; butterscotch
Soups	Bouillon; broth; broth-based soups	Cream soups and chowders; dehydrated soup mixes made with milk products
Miscellaneous	Herbs and spices; salt and pepper; whey solids; plain tortilla or potato chips; salsa; mustard; ketchup; pickles	Medications or vitamin/mineral supplements that contain lactose as a filler; sugar substitutes with lactose added

References

Chronic Diarrhea

1. American Gastroenterological Association medical position statement: Guidelines for the evaluation and management of chronic diarrhea. *Gastroenterology*. 1999 June;116, (6): 1461-1463.

2. Bonis PA, LaMont JT. Approach to the adult with chronic diarrhea in developed countries. *UpToDate®*. Topic updated June 7, 2011.

3. Fine KD, Schiller LR. AGA Technical Review on the Evaluation and Management of Chronic Diarrhea. *Gastroenterology*. 1999 July; 116 (6): 1464-1486.

4. http://www.pdrhealth.com/drug_info/nmdrugprofiles/nutsupdrugs/pro_0034.shtml

5. http://www.mdanderson.org/transcripts/POE-Diarrhea-Multiple-Causes-Bisanz.htm

6. Bisanz A, Tucker AM, Amin DM, Patel D, Calderon BB, Joseph NM, Curry EA 3rd. Summary of the causative and treatment factors of diarrhea and the use of a diarrhea assessment and treatment tool to improve patient outcomes. *Gastroenterol Nurs*. 2010 Jul-Aug;33(4):268-81; quiz 282-3.

7. http://www.nutritioncaremanual.org. Accessed March 16, 2011.

8. Zied, Elisa. *Nutrition at Your Fingertips*. The Stonesong Press; 2009.

9. Kelly DG, Nadeu J. Oral Rehydration Solution: A "Low-Tech" Oft Neglected Therapy. *Practical Gastroenterology*. October 2004.

10. Oral Rehydration Therapy Fact Sheet. Cera Products, Inc. 2010.

11. http://www.med.unc.edu/ibs/files/educational-gi-handouts/IBS%20and%20Hormones.pdf

12. Hofmann AF. Chronic diarrhea caused by idiopathic bile acid malabsorption: an explanation at last. *Expert Rev Gastroenterol Hepatol.* 2009*b*; 3: 461-464.

13. Office of Dietary Supplements. *National Institutes of Health.* http://ods.od.nih.gov/factsheets/list-all/. Accessed July 10, 2012.

14. Norman K, Kirchner H, Lochs H, Pirlich M. Malnutrition affects quality of life in gastroenterology patients. *World J Gastroenterol.* 2006; 12(21): 3380-3385.

Probiotics and Prebiotics

15. Sartor RB. Probiotics for gastrointestinal diseases. *UpToDate®*. Topic updated January 30, 2013.

16. http://www.consumerlab.com/news/probiotics-review/2_9_2012/

17. http://www.isapp.net/docs/Consumer_Guidelines_final.pdf Accessed October 12, 2012.

18. Hempel S, et al. Probiotics for the Prevention and Treatment of Antibiotic-Associated Diarrhea. A Systematic Review and Meta-analysis. *JAMA.* 2012;307(18):1959-1969.

19. Probiotics and prebiotics. May 2008. World Gastroenterology Organisation Practice Guideline. Available at: http://www.worldgastroenterology.org/assets/downloads/en/pdf/guidel ines/19_probiotics_prebiotics.pdf Accessed: October 20, 2011

20. Jenkins B, Holsten S, Bengmark S, Martindale R. Probiotics: a practical review of their role in specific clinical scenarios. *Nutr Clin Prac.* 2005;20:262-270.

21. Floch MH, Hong-Curtiss J. Probiotics and functional foods in gastrointestinal disorders. *Current Treatment Options in Gastroenterology.* 2002, 5:311-321.

22. Georgetown University Medical Center. Kefir, Although Rich In Probiotics, Didn't Prevent Diarrhea In Children Using Antibiotics. *ScienceDaily*, 4 August 2009.

23. http://www.usprobiotics.org Accessed October 15, 2012.

24. http://www.gutmicrobiotawatch.org. Accessed February 20, 2013.

25. http://www.gastro.org/patient-center/brochure_Probiotics.pdf. Accessed October 17, 2012.

Irritable Bowel Syndrome

26. American College of Gastroenterology IBS Task Force. An Evidence-based Position Statement on the Management of Irritable Bowel Syndrome. *Am J Gastroenterology*. 2009; 104:S1-S35.

27. Houghton LA, Lea R, Jackson N, Whorwell PJ. The menstrual cycle affects rectal sensitivity in patients with irritable bowel syndrome but not healthy volunteers. *GUT*. 2002;50:471-74.

28. Pimentel M, Soffer EE, Chow EJ, et al. Lower frequency of MMC is found in IBS subjects with abnormal lactulose breath test, suggesting bacterial overgrowth. *Dig Dis Sci*, 2002;47:2639-2643.

29. Ruepert L, Quartero AO, de Wit NJ, et al. Bulking agents, antispasmodics and antidepressants for the treatment of irritable bowel syndrome. *Cochrane Database Syst Rev*. Accessed August 10, 2011.

30. Eswaran S, Tack J, Chey WD. Food: The Forgotten Factor in the Irritable Bowel Syndrome. *Gastroenterol Clin N Am*. 40 (2011) 141–162.

31. Thompson, WG, Creed, F, Drossman, DA, Mazzaca, G. Functional bowel disorders and chronic abdominal pain. *Gastroenterol Int* 1992; 5:75.

32. Wald A. Treatment of irritable bowel syndrome. *UpToDate®*. Topic updated December 20, 2012.

FODMAPs

33. Barrett JS, Gibson PR. Clinical ramifications of malabsorption of fructose and other short-chain carbohydrates. *Pract. Gastroenterol.* 2007; 31:51-65.

34. Catsos P. *IBS—Free at Last! Change Your Carbs, Change Your Life*. Portland (ME): Pond Cove Press; 2012.

35. http://www.ibsfree.net/ (Patsy Catsos' website with practical tips for following the FODMAPS diet.)

36. Gearry RB, Irving PM, Barrett JS, Nathan D, Shepherd SJ, Gibson PR. Reduction of dietary FODMAPs improves abdominal symptoms in patients with inflammatory bowel disease—a pilot study. *J. Crohns Colitis* 2009;3: 8–14.

37. Gibson PR, Shepherd SJ. Evidence-based Dietary Management of Functional Gastrointestinal Symptoms: The FODMAP Approach. *J Gastroenterol Hepatol.* 2010;25(2):252-258.

38. Scarlata K. The FODMAPs approach—Minimize consumption of Fermentable Carbs to Manage Functional Gut Disorder. *Today's Dietitian.* Vol 12 Number 9 p 30.

39. Shepherd SJ, Gibson PR. Fructose malabsorption and symptoms of irritable bowel syndrome: guidelines for effective dietary management. *J. Am. Diet. Assoc.* 2006; 106:1631-9.

40. Shepherd SJ, Parker FJ, Muir JG, Gibson PR. Dietary Triggers of abdominal symptoms in patients with irritable bowel syndrome: randomised placebo-controlled evidence. *Clin Gastroenterol. Hepatol.* 2008; 6:765-71.

41. Eswaran S, Tack J, Chey W. Food: The Forgotten Factor in the Irritable Bowel Syndrome. *Gastroenterol Clin N Am.* 40 (2011) 141–162.

42. Muir JG, Shepherd SJ, Rosella O, Rose, R, Barrett JS, and Gibson PR. Fructan and Free Fructose Content of Common Australian Vegetables and Fruit. *J. Agric. Food Chem.* 2007;55(16), 6619-6627.

43. Heizer WD, Southern S, McGovern S. The Role of Diet in Symptoms of Irritable Bowel Syndrome in Adults: A Narrative Review. *J Am Diet Assoc.* 2009; 109:1204-1214.

44. Scarlatta, K. *The Complete Idiot's Guide to Eating Well for IB.* Alpha, 2010.

45. Shepherd S. *The Low-FODMAP Diet; Fructose Malabsorption Shopping Guide.* 5th ed. Shepherd Works Pty Ltd, 2010.

46. http://shepherdworks.com.au/disease-information/low-fodmap-diet. Accessed May 24, 2012.

Celiac Disease

47. Rubio-Tapia A, Ludvigsson JF, Brantner TL, et al. The prevalence of celiac disease in the United States. *Am J Gastroenterol.* 2012 Oct; 107 (10):1538-44.

48. Sapone, et al. Divergence of gut permeability and mucosal immune gene expression in two gluten-associated conditions: celiac disease and gluten sensitivity. *BMC Medicine.* 2011, 9:23.

49. Fasano A. Surprises from Celiac Disease. *Scientific American.* Aug 2009: 54-61.

50. Fasano A. Zonulin and Its Regulation of Intestinal Barrier Function: The Biological Door to Inflammation, Autoimmunity, and Cancer. *Physio Rev.* 2011; 91:151-175.

Food Allergy and Intolerance

51. http://www.fda.gov/food/resourcesforyou/consumers/ucm079311.htm Accessed December 10, 2012.

52. http://www.foodallergy.org/files/FoodAllergyFactsandStatistics.pdf Accessed December 12, 2012.

53. Wang J. Sampson HA. Food allergy: recent advances in pathophysiology and treatment. *Allergy Asthma Immunol Res.* 2009 October; 1(1): 19–29.

54. Joneja, Janice Vickerstaff. *Dealing with Food Allergies: a practical guide to detecting culprit foods and eating a healthy, enjoyable diet*. Bull Publishing Company. Boulder, Colorado, 2003.

55. Simren M, Stotzer P-O. Use and abuse of hydrogen breath tests. *Gut.* 2006;55:297–303.

56. Lactose Intolerance. Scientific Status Report. Dairy Research Institute. 2011.

57. U.S. Department of Agriculture, Agricultural Research Service. 2011. USDA National Nutrient Database for Standard Reference, Release 24. Nutrient Data Laboratory Home Page, http://www.ars.usda.gov/ba/bhnrc/ndl. Accessed December 1, 2011.

58. http://www.lactaid.com/products-home#Calcium_Enriched_Fat_Free. Accessed December 1, 2011.

59. http://silksoymilk.com/nutriInfo/PlainNATQuart.htm. Accessed December 1, 2011.

60. http://nutritiondata.self.com/facts-C00001-01c200_B0003s1m110701000K060105050000020K00Hempqq0Milkqq0qq8Hempqq0Blissqq0originalqq0flavorqq9.html. Accessed December 1, 2011.

Small Intestinal Bacterial Overgrowth (SIBO)

61. Teo M, Chung S, Chitti L, et al. Small bowel bacterial overgrowth is a common cause of chronic diarrhea. *J Gastro Hepatol*. 2004;19:904-909.

62. Dukowicz AC. Lacy BE. Levine GM. Small Intestinal Bacterial Overgrowth: A Comprehensive Review. *Gastroenterology and Hepatology* Volume 3, Issue 2 February 2007: 112-122.

63. Zaidel O. Lin HC. Uninvited Guests: The Impact of Small Intestinal Bacterial Overgrowth on Nutritional Status. *Practical Gastroenterology*. Jul 2003; 7: 27-34.

64. DiBaise JK. Nutritional Consequences of Small Intestinal Bacterial Overgrowth. *Practical Gastroenterology*. Dec 2008; 69: 15-28.

65. Pimentel D. *A New IBS Solution*. Sherman Oaks, CA: Health Point Press; 2006.

Other

66. Lewis SJ, Heaton KW. Stool form scale as a useful guide to intestinal transit time. *Scand. J. Gastroenterol.* 1997; 32 (9): 920–4.

67. http://www.nlm.nih.gov/medlineplus/ency/article/000347.htm. Accessed January 3, 2013.

68. http://www.iom.edu/Reports/2006/Dietary-Reference-Intakes-Essential-Guide-Nutrient-Requirements.aspx Accessed December 7, 2012.

69. Sullivan SN, Wong C. Runners' diarrhea. Different patterns and associated factors. *J Clin Gastroenterol*. 1992;14(2):101-104.

70. Clausen JP. Effect of physical training on cardiovascular adjustments to exercise in man. *Physiol Rev*. 1977;57(4):779-815.

Web Resources

IBS and Functional Bowel Disorders

- https://www.inspire.com/groups/agmd-gi-motility/about/
  Association of Gastrointestinal Motility Disorders, Inc. (AGMD)

- http://www.iffgd.org/
  International Foundation for Functional Gastrointestinal Disorders (IFFGD)

- http://www.ibsgroup.org/
  Irritable Bowel Syndrome Self Help and Support Group

Inflammatory Bowel Disease

- http://www.ccfa.org/about/?LMI=0
  Crohn's and Colitis Foundation of America (CCFA)

- https://www.ecco-ibd.eu/
  European Crohn's and Colitis Organisation (ECCO)

Celiac Disease

- http://www.gluten.net/
  Gluten Intolerance Group (GIG)

- http://www.csaceliacs.org
  Celiac Sprue Association (CSA)

- http://www.celiac.org
  Celiac Disease Foundation (CDF)

- www.celiacdiseasecenter.columbia.edu

- www.celiaccenter.org
  The University of Maryland Center for Celiac Research

- http://www.celiacnow.org
  Beth Israel Deaconess Medical Center, a teaching hospital of Harvard Medical School

- http://www.celiac.com

Food Allergies
- http://www.foodallergy.org
  The Food Allergy and Anaphylaxis Network (FAAN)

- http://www.aaaai.org
  American Academy of Allergy Asthma and Immunology (AAAAI)

General Gastrointestinal Resources
- http://digestive.niddk.nih.gov/index.aspx
  National Digestive Diseases Information Clearinghouse (NDDIC)

- http://www.gastro.org/
  American Gastroenterological Association (AGA)

- http://gi.org/
  American College of Gastroenterology (ACG)

- http://badgut.org
  Canadian Society of Gastrointestinal Research

- http://www.digestivedistress.com/our-mission
  The Gastroparesis and Dysmotilities Association

- http://www.practicalgastro.com/index.html
  Practical Gastroenterology — a peer-reviewed professional medical journal focused on the diagnosis and management of digestive diseases

General Nutrition
- http://www.eatright.org
  Academy of Nutrition and Dietetics (formerly the American Dietetic Association). Use this site to find a registered dietitian near you.

- http://www.nutrition411.com/

About the Author

Niki Strealy, RD, LD received her bachelor's degree in nutrition and food management from Oregon State University and completed a dietetic internship at Vanderbilt University Medical Center. She has worked as a registered dietitian since 1996, providing nutrition counseling in both hospital and outpatient clinics. Her specialty is gastrointestinal diseases and disorders. The Oregon Dietetic Association named her the "Recognized Young Dietitian of the Year" in 2000.

She lives in Portland, Oregon with her husband, three favorite kids, and flock of chickens. She enjoys running, playing and watching soccer, spending time with family and friends, camping, photography, gardening, scrapbooking, watching Oregon State football, public speaking, and talking about her favorite subject, diarrhea.

Index

Funny jokes that came up during the writing of this book:

- "I write when I can. It comes in *spurts*."
- "Doing all this research has me *running* around."
- "If I make a mistake, I want to *rectify* it before it's finished."
- "Wow, you can't stop talking about your book. You have diarrhea of the mouth."
- "The *bottom* line is: I just have to finish writing it."
- "Mom, I have diarrhea... dot com." (by my 5 year old daughter)

Books titles I loved, but weren't appropriate for this book:

- D—Tools from the Diarrhea Dietitian
- Every Party has a Pooper. A dietitian's guide to nutrition for chronic diarrhea
- Dear Diarrhea. It's Not You. It's Me. A dietitian's guide to dumping chronic diarrhea for good
- How to Skirt the Squirts
- Taming the Flaming Fury of Chronic Diarrhea
- Diarrhea, Diarrhea, I Hope to Never See Ya
- What a Blast—the Diarrhea Survival Guide
- How to Deal with the Big D—What you eat makes the difference
- Chronic Diarrhea Guidebook
- Hope of Healing Through Nutrition
- The Diarrhea Dilemma
- Revealing the Bowel Mysteries of Chronic Diarrhea
- Stop the Runs: Words of Wisdom from the Diarrhea Dietitian
- Eating Secrets from the Diarrhea Dietitian
- Stop Running... Advice from the Diarrhea Dietitian
- The Diarrhea Dietitian: A Complete Guidebook to Coping with the Big D
- The Diarrhea Dietitian: Empowering You to Dump the Big D for Good

36204315R00139

Made in the USA
Lexington, KY
10 October 2014